THE LECTIN

FREE

COOKBOOK

Alice Liberti

damages, or monetary loss due to the information herein, either directly or indirectly.

Respective authors own all copyrights not held by the publisher.

The information herein is offered for informational purposes solely, and is universal as so. The presentation of the information is without contract or any type of guarantee assurance.

The trademarks that are used are without any consent, and the publication of the trademark is without permission or backing by the trademark owner. All trademarks and brands within this book are for clarifying purposes only and are the owned by the owners themselves, not affiliated with this document.

Table of Contents

- HEARTY SPINACH BEEF FRITTATA RECIPE
- OATMEAL COTTAGE CHEESE BANANA PANCAKES
- PALEO BREAKFAST CASSEROLE
- BREAKFAST PIZZA
- KALE SALAD WITH MUSHROOM OMELET RECIPE
- PALEO BREAKFAST PORRIDGE RECIPE
- PALEO CINNAMON RAISIN BAGELS
- PANCAKE BUNS
- EGG PATTY
- PALEO AND KETO EGG MUFFIN RECIPE
- PEACH COBBLER OATMEAL
- PUMPKIN PIE OATMEAL RECIPE
- GLUTEN-FREE VEGAN RASPBERRY ALMOND SQUARES
- PALEO RASPBERRY POP TARTS
- RAW APPLE-CINNAMON & CHIA BREAKFAST BOWL
- SAGE CHICKEN BREAKFAST PATTIES RECIPE
- SHAKSHUKA
- 3-INGREDIENT BANANA PUDDING RECIPE
- TURKEY SAUSAGE, BROCCOLI & TOMATO CRUSTLESS QUICHE
- TURMERIC EGGS RECIPE
- VANILLA CHIA PUDDING RECIPE
- VEGGIE QUICHE CUPS TO-GO
- 2 MINUTE PALEO PORRIDGE
- SHEET PAN CLASSIC BREAKFAST
- MAPLE PECAN GRAIN-FREE GRANOLA
- GRAIN-FREE GRANOLA

- AVOCADO SWEET POTATO TOAST WITH POACHED EGG
- MUSHROOM RISOTTO WITH CAULIFLOWER RICE
- THAI RED CURRY CHICKEN
- ROASTED CAULIFLOWER STEAKS WITH LEMON DILL TAHINI SAUCE
- BASIL AND ARTICHOKE SHIRATAKI FETTUCCINE PASTA
- GLUTEN-FREE VEGAN CARROT "HOT DOG"
- CILANTRO PESTO SWEET POTATO SALAD
- TURMERIC AND BLACK PEPPERCORN SESAME SEED CRACKERS
- VEGAN CREAM OF MUSHROOM SOUP
- SPICY TURMERIC OVEN-BAKED SWEET POTATO FRIES
- CLASSIC HUMMUS
- OVEN-BAKED "FRIED" ARTICHOKES
- CHIMICHURRI SAUCE
- CHOCOLATE AVOCADO PUDDING
- SWEET POTATO HUMMUS
- LEMON DILL AVOCADO DRESSING
- RAW CACAO AND RASPBERRY MOUSSE CAKES
- CHOCOLATE CAULIFLOWER NICE CREAM SMOOTHIE BOWL
- RAW NO-BAKE BLACK FOREST BARS
- VEGAN RASPBERRY AND CHOCOLATE ICE CREAM SQUARES
- VEGAN DRIED BLUEBERRY PROTEIN ENERGY BALLS

- VEGAN CHOCOLATE DIPPED CHERRIES
- CHOCOLATE PISTACHIO FUDGE CUPS WITH SEA SALT
- VEGAN CHOCOLATE COVERED STRAWBERRY TRUFFLES
- VEGAN "CHEESY" BROCCOLI BITES
- VEGAN CHILLED MIXED BERRY AND MINT SOUP
- VEGAN LEMON MOUSSE TARTS
- VEGAN VANILLA BEAN ICE CREAM
- ALMOND BUTTER SWIRL, CHOCOLATE AVOCADO ICE CREAM
- VEGAN STRAWBERRY MOUSSE
- HEALTHY HONEY MUSTARD DRESSING
- VEGAN CHOCOLATE COVERED TURTLES
- VEGAN TAHINI BROWNIE TRUFFLES
- VEGAN TACO "MEAT"
- VEGAN CHOCOLATE AVOCADO FROSTING
- VEGAN CACAO ALMOND BALLS
- VEGAN CARAMEL SAUCE
- VEGAN CILANTRO AND LIME CAULIFLOWER RICE
- VEGAN SPINACH PESTO
- SHIRATAKI ANGEL HAIR PASTA WITH CREAMY CHIPOTLE AVOCADO SAUCE
- CARROT APPLE AND CELERY JUICE
- VEGAN FLOURLESS "CHEESY" GARLIC BREADSTICKS
- VEGAN FRESH HERB AND TAHINI PESTO
- VEGAN SWEET POTATO AND PECAN BALLS

- CHIPOTLE ALMOND STUFFED BRUSSELS SPROUTS
- VEGAN BASIL PESTO AND CAULIFLOWER RICE DIP
- VEGAN CHOCOLATE AVOCADO PISTACHIO TRUFFLES
- VEGAN PECAN PIE TRUFFLES
- VEGAN CREAM OF ASPARAGUS SOUP

Introductions

I make sound sans lectin formulas that are straightforward and simple to make and they're perfect eating, crude, veggie lover, sans gluten, sans dairy, sans egg, without grain, flourless, paleo, refined sans sugar and some no-heat as well! Additionally, I have more than 450+ clean eating, sans gluten and vegetarian formulas on my site and am at present during the time spent experiencing them all to name the ones that are 100% without lectin veggie lover, and also, making formula adjustments to existing formulas to make them sans lectin vegetarian.

What is the lectin-free diet?

without lectin eat less. He is a previous heart specialist who changed his concentration to nourishment and supplement-based pharmaceutical.

lectins It was portrayed as the fundamental risk found in the American eating regimen. Accordingly, he has composed a book that gives data on the most proficient method to maintain a strategic distance from lectins, elective sustenance decisions, and formulas.

Plan enables individuals to enhance their wellbeing and lessen their body weight. The arrangement additionally incorporates supplements built up that are sold under the brand.

What are lectins?

Undercooked red kidney beans may cause extreme queasiness, the runs, and regurgitating because of a lectin called phytohemagglutinin.

Lectins are a kind of protein that, in people, may enable cells to communicate with each other. A few researchers likewise trust that lectins give a type of resistance in plants to fend off creepy crawlies.

These proteins additionally contain nitrogen, which is required for plants to develop. While numerous parts of plants contain lectins, the seed is the part that individuals eat regularly.

Lectins may affect wellbeing in various courses, extending from processing to endless infection chance. They have been appeared to make red platelets bunch together.

Grain Free Applesauce Pancakes

Ingredients:

- 2 - eggs
- 1/3 - cup applesauce, unsweetened
- ¼ - cup almond meal
- ½ - teaspoon baking powder
- ¼ - teaspoon vanilla extract
- ½ - tablespoon maple syrup/honey/agave nectar

Instructions:

1. Whisk 2 eggs in a little bowl. At that point transfer in fruit purée, maple syrup, and vanilla concentrate.
2. Include almond feast and heating powder and mix until blended.
3. Splash a container with coconut oil shower or nonstick cooking shower and warmth to low/medium. Once the skillet is totally warmed. Spoon in roughly 3 tablespoons of hitter.
4. Let cook for around 3-4 minutes on the principal side, or till firm adequate to flip. You'll have to transport quick while flipping with a spatula.
5. Cook the second one side for cycle 2-3 mins or till totally cooked. Rehash three more circumstances.

Autumn Sweet Potato Hash

Ingredients:

- 2 - links Spicy Italian Sausage, casing removed
- 2 - sweet potatoes, peeled and diced into tiny cubes
- 1 - small onion, diced
- 1 - red bell pepper, cored and seeded, and diced
- Salt
- Black pepper
- Paprika (Pinch)
- onion powder (Pinch)
- garlic powder (Pinch)
- Italian seasoning (Pinch)
- 2 - teaspoons chopped fresh flat-leaf parsley
- 1 - green onion, chopped
- ¼ - cup grated asiago cheese

Instructions:

1. Place an expansive non-stick sauté container over medium-high warmth; once hot, disintegrate the zesty frankfurter into the skillet permitting it remain moderately thick, and dark colored it for a few minutes.
2. Next, include into the dish the onion and the red ringer pepper, and sauté those with the hotdog for a couple of minutes until brilliant dark colored (if somewhat more

oil is required, include a sprinkle of olive oil); include a squeeze or two of salt and naturally ground dark pepper, the squeeze of paprika, onion powder, garlic powder and Italian flavoring, and blend to consolidate; include the diced sweet potato, mix, and cook everything until the point when it begins to caramelize and diminish somewhat, secured, for around 10-12 minutes, mixing at times.

3. Complete the hash by including the cleaved parsley and green onion, and overlay those in; spoon the hash into dishes or plates, and best with the ground asiago cheddar; present with a fricasseed egg, if wanted

Avocado Bacon and Eggs

Ingredients:

- 1 - medium Avocado
- 2 - eggs
- 1 - piece of cooked bacon
- 1 - TB of low-fat cheese
- pinch of salt

Instructions:

1. Preheat stove to 425.
2. Start by slicing the avocado down the middle and expelling the pit.
3. With a spoon, scoop out a portion of the avocado so it's a bit greater than your egg and yolk. Place in a biscuit container to keep the avocado stable while cooking.
4. Break your egg and add it to within your avocado. Sprinkle a little cheddar on top with a squeeze of salt. Top with cooked bacon

Baked Pears with Walnuts and Honey

Ingredients:

- 2 - large ripe pears
- ¼ - tsp ground cinnamon
- 2 - tsp honey
- ¼ - cup crushed walnuts
- yogurt or frozen yogurt

Instructions:

1. Preheat the broiler to 350°F.
2. Cut the pears down the middle and place on a heating sheet (I cut a bit off the opposite end so they sat upright).
3. Utilizing an estimating spoon or melon hotshot, scoop out the seeds.
4. Sprinkle with cinnamon, top with walnuts and shower ½ teaspoon nectar over every one.
5. Heat in the stove 30 minutes. Evacuate, let cool and appreciate!

Baked Quinoa with Apples Recipe

Ingredients:

- ½ - cup quinoa
- 1 - cup water
- 2 - eggs
- 5 - tablespoons applesauce
- pinch of sea salt
- ¼ - teaspoon cinnamon
- 2 - teaspoons chopped pecans
- ¾ - cup apple
- 1 - teaspoon honey

Instructions:

1. Bubble Water at that point include Quinoa and stew for 10-15 mins.
2. Fill broiler safe bowl, include Eggs, Apple Sauce, Salt and Cinnamon and sear on low in stove for 7 mins.
3. Top with Pecans, Apple and Honey

Blueberry Oatmeal Pancakes

Ingredients:

- 1 - tablespoon freshly ground flaxseed meal
- 3 - tablespoons warm water
- ½ - cup brown rice flour
- ½ - cup quick cooking oats
- 1 - tablespoon agave nectar
- 1 - teaspoon baking powder
- ½ - teaspoon baking soda
- ½ - teaspoon salt
- 1 - teaspoon lemon juice
- ¾ - cup almond milk
- 1 - teaspoon vanilla extract
- 1 - tablespoon coconut oil, melted
- 1 - cup blueberries
- blueberry chia jam, to serve
- maple syrup, to serve

Instructions:

1. integrate the tablespoon of flaxseed supper and 3 tablespoons heat water and positioned aside till gooey, relatively like egg whites.

2. In an estimating glass, consist of 1 teaspoon lemon squeeze at that factor give up off with almond drain to make 3/4 field. blend and placed aside till soured.
3. In a blender, encompass oats and mix unexpectedly until nearly frames a flour. consist of ultimate fixings, aside from blueberries, and mix until smooth.
4. warmth a lightly oiled skillet or iron over medium warmth. Spoon flapjack hitter on, round 1/four area for every hotcake, and location round five-7 blueberries to finish the whole lot. cook dinner till the thing while bubbles form and burst at first appearance. turn with a spatula and press right down to cook dinner equitably. cook dinner around three extra mins, or until cooked thru. gift with blueberry chia stick and maple syrup.

Breakfast Quesadilla Recipe

Ingredients:

- 1 - peach, peeled and diced
- 1 - pear, peeled and diced
- ¼ - cup sprouted almond butter
- cinnamon to taste
- 1 - tablespoon coconut oil
- 1 - tablespoon raw honey
- 4 - brown rice, grain less or Ezekiel tortillas

Instructions:

1. On the focal point of the tortilla, spread almond margarine and best it with the diced peaches and pears. Shower the natural product with nectar and sprinkle cinnamon to finish everything. Place a second tortilla to finish everything.
2. In an expansive skillet over medium warmth, dissolve coconut oil or spread.
3. Place quesadilla in the skillet, flipping once, until the point that the two sides are brilliant darker and fresh. Rehash with outstanding tortillas.
4. Sprinkle with nectar and serve.

Breakfast Salmon Egg Bake Recipe

Ingredients:

- 2 - tablespoons ghee
- 1 - medium onion, thinly sliced crosswise
- 8 - large eggs
- 1 - cup red, yellow and/or orange peppers, chopped
- 1 - cup kefir
- 1 - cup mushrooms
- 1 - tablespoons chopped fresh dill
- Sea Salt and black pepper
- 1 - teaspoon nutmeg
- 6 - ounces smoked wild caught Alaskan salmon, skin removed and roughly broken into 1/2-inch pieces
- ¾ - cup goat cheese, crumbled

Instructions:

1. Preheat grill to 350 levels F
2. Diminish the ghee in a ten-inch sauté dish over medium-high warmth. Incorporate the onion and peppers and cook, mixing every so often, till touchy and turning translucent, around three mins. Incorporate the mushrooms and cook supper until appeased and amazingly caramelized, some other three to four minutes. Oust the container from the glow.

3. Spread blend with ghee over base of lubed dish
4. Spread salmon segments over onion mix
5. Beat the eggs in a medium bowl/container with the kefir, 1 tbsp of the dill, ¼ tsp. Salt, ¼ tsp. Pepper, and the nutmeg.
6. Pour egg blend over onion blend
7. Warmth for 35-40 mins
8. Sprinkle goat cheddar over pleasant and serve.

Broiled Grapefruit

Ingredients:

- honey

- grapefruit

- ground ginger (ground cinnamon is a good substitute or addition)

- Banana slices (strawberries would be nice too) optional

Instructions:

1. Plan stove for searing. Position broiler rack to finish everything.
2. Cut grapefruit(s) into equal parts. Utilizing a little serrated blade or grapefruit cut, extricate the grapefruit segments from the film. Place the grapefruit parts on a preparing sheet or shallow heating container.
3. Sprinkle grapefruit parts with nectar. Place banana cuts to finish everything and flip once to coat the two sides with nectar. Residue with ground ginger (as well as cinnamon).
4. Place under oven until the point that percolating and marginally sautéed in spots, around 4 to 6 minutes. Watch out for amid cooking to abstain from consuming.
5. Serve warm.

Buffalo Chicken Egg Muffins

Ingredients:

- ¾ - lb. skin on Chicken Thigh, boneless, skinless (or breast meat)
- ½ - tsp Garlic Powder
- 1 - tsp Salt and Pepper, to taste, + 1 tsp
- ¼ - cup Tessemae's Hot Sauce / Wing Sauce, + 2 Tbsp (or other with clean ingredients)
- 6 - Eggs, whisked
- 2 - Tbsp Green Onion, sliced

Instructions:

1. Preheat the range to 425.
2. On a getting ready skillet, orchestrate the bird thighs and season with garlic, ocean salt, and dark pepper. Prepare for 25 minutes or till cooked through.
3. Place the cooked hen thighs into an extensive mixing dish and shred with two forks. Pour the wing sauce over the fowl and hurl to consolidate and put it aside.
4. In a little blending dish, whisk the eggs, wing sauce, inexperienced onion, ocean salt, and dark pepper.
5. Empty the egg combination into fabric glass lined (those are the main form of liners I prescribe as nothing sticks to them, ensured!) biscuit tins to fill them round midway. Tenderly spoon round 2oz of the destroyed bird into every biscuit container so it is similarly

conveyed. Serve any extra bird nearby the cooked biscuits.

6. Prepare for roughly half-hour or till the factor that the biscuits rise and come to be splendid dark colored around the edges.

Chicken Butternut Squash Hazelnut Mash

Ingredients:

- 1 - medium (800g) butternut squash, cut in half and seeds removed

- 2 - medium (200g each) boneless skinless chicken breasts

- A sprinkle of Himalayan or fine sea salt

- Few grinds freshly cracked pepper

- The juice of one orange

- The juice of one orange

- 6 - cups fresh baby spinach leaves, chopped

- 50g - hazelnuts, crushed

- ¼ - cup coconut milk or cream

- ½ - tsp chai spice*

Instructions:

1. Preheat your stove to 350F.
2. Sprinkle the butternut squash parts with a bit of salt and pepper. Place them look down in a shallow warming dish adequately immense to oblige the two sections and also the chicken chests.
3. Place the chicken chests in a comparable compartment with the squash and sprinkle them too with some salt and pepper. (if in spite of all that you have space available, for what reason not acknowledge this open way to cook two or three more chests? That way you'll end up with some wonderful staying cooked chicken in the cooler, and that is for the most part SO beneficial to have!)
4. Squash the juice of the orange over the chicken chests, leave the empty orange shells in the dish and cover with frustrate.
5. Place that in the stove and cook for 30-35 minutes, until the point when the squash is decent and delicate and the chicken is cooked through; expel thwart and forget to cool for a couple of minutes.
6. While that is going on, add the spinach to a substantial non-stick skillet, and cook until the point that simply withered, around 2-3 minutes. On the other hand, you could likewise wither the spinach by popping it in the microwave for 1 or 2 minutes.
7. While the spinach is shriveling, toast the pulverized hazelnuts in a little, dry skillet over medium warmth.
8. By at that point, the chicken and squash ought to be sufficiently cool to deal with; shred the chicken into nibble estimate pieces and place them in a substantial blending dish. Utilizing a spoon, scoop out the substance from the squash and add that to the held chicken. Include spinach, hazelnuts, coconut cream and chai flavor and blend gently until the point that all around joined.
9. Separation this blend between 2 stove safe dishes and place under the oven until the best takes a decent brilliant hue.
10. Trimming with more pounded hazelnuts and coconut cream, if wanted.

Cauliflower Tortillas

Ingredients:

- ¾ - head cauliflower
- 2 - large eggs
- ¼ - cup chopped fresh cilantro
- juice from ½ lime (add the zest too if you want more of a lime flavor)
- salt and pepper, to taste

Instructions:

1. Preheat the range to 375 ranges F. besides line a getting equipped sheet with material paper.
2. Trim the cauliflower, cut it into little, uniform pieces, and pulse in a sustenance processor in bunches until the point which you get a couscous-like consistency. The finely riced cauliflower needs to make round 2 holders stuffed.
3. location the cauliflower in a microwave-safe bowl and microwave for 2 mins, through then combination and microwave again for an extra 2 minutes. region the cauliflower in an exceptional cheesecloth or thin dishtowel and pound out anyway a good deal liquid as might be regular, being careful in order not to deplete yourself. Dishwashing gloves are prescribed as it's far outstandingly warm.
4. In a medium bowl, whisk the eggs. Include cauliflower, cilantro, lime, salt, and pepper. Blend until the point

when all around consolidated. Utilize your hands to shape 6 little "tortillas" on the material paper.

5. Heat for 10 minutes, deliberately flip every tortilla and come back to the stove for an extra 5 to 7 minutes, or until totally set. Place tortillas on a wire rack to cool somewhat.

6. Warmth a medium-sized skillet on medium. Place a prepared tortilla in the skillet, pushing down marginally, and dark colored for 1 to 2 minutes on each side. Rehash with residual tortillas.

Chocolate Covered Cherry Kefir Smoothie

Ingredients:

- 2 - cups milk kefir
- ¾ - cup frozen cherries
- 4 - TBSP honey, maple syrup or a sprinkle of stevia
- 1/3 - cup of soy free chocolate chips

Instructions:

1. Put all fixings (with the exception of a little bunch of chocolate chips) in an excellent blender and blender and mix until smooth. Fill glasses and afterward hack remaining chocolate chips into modest pieces and sprinkle over the smoothie. Appreciate!
2. Do you have a most adored kefir smoothie recipe? I would love to see the recipe! An obligation of appreciation is all together to make a trek and let me know how you like this one!

Classic (Paleo) Diner-Style Home Fries

Ingredients:

- 1 - pound organic potatoes, peeled and cut into ½ -inch cubes
- 1 - teaspoon salt
- 1 - medium onion, finely diced (LIKE 1 cup)
- ½ - tablespoon plus 2 tablespoons cooking fat (coconut oil, lard, duck fat)
- 1 - teaspoon paprika
- ½ - teaspoon chili powder
- ¼ - teaspoon salt
- ¼ - teaspoon ground black pepper
- ¼ - cup fresh parsley leaves, minced (LIKE 1 tablespoon)

Instructions:

1. Place diced potatoes and salt in a pan, cover with ½ inch water, and place over high warmth. At the point when the water starts to bubble, around 6-8 minutes, check the potatoes to check whether they're sufficiently delicate to penetrate with a fork. On the off chance that yes, deplete them altogether in a colander.
2. In the meantime, while the potatoes are cooking, warm an expansive skillet over medium-high warmth, around 3 minutes. Add fat and enable it to soften. Hurl the onion in the skillet and sauté, mixing as often as

possible with a wooden spoon. Cook until pleasantly caramelized, around 8-10 minutes. Exchange the onion to a little bowl and restore the skillet to the warmth.

3. Add 2 tablespoons coconut oil to the skillet and enable the dish to get hot, around 2 minutes. Include the potato 3D squares, shaking the skillet to influence an even, single to layer. Cook the spuds without blending until the point when the 3D squares are brilliant dark colored on the base, around 5 minutes, at that point painstakingly flip them with a huge spatula and make another single layer. Rehash this procedure until the point that the shapes are sautéed on most sides, around 15 minutes.

4. At the point when the potatoes are solid, include the onions, paprika, stew powder, salt, and pepper to the skillet. Mix to mix and warmth through. Expel the home fries from the warmth, blend in the parsley, and serve quickly.

Easy Blueberry Jam

Ingredients:

- 2 - cups fresh organic
  blueberries
- 2 - tablespoons raw honey
- 2 - tablespoons lemon juice
- 2 - tablespoons chia seeds

Instructions:

1. Coat blueberries with crude nectar
2. Exchange covered blueberries to a pot and include lemon juice
3. Warmth over medium/low warmth until the point when blueberries are delicate and percolating (5 minutes)
4. Gently crush blueberries and lessen warm marginally
5. Include chia seeds and blend to consolidate
6. Take warm back to medium/low and let bubble (yet not consume) until the point that stick thickens (another 5 or so minutes)
7. Turn warm off and let cool for 5-10 minutes before exchanging to containers
8. Store in ice chest for up to 2 weeks

Eggs Baked in Portobello Mushrooms

Ingredients:

- 4 - large portobello mushrooms, stem removed, wiped clean
- Olive oil spray
- ½ - teaspoon kosher salt, divided
- ½ - teaspoon black pepper, divided
- ½ - teaspoon garlic powder
- 4 - medium eggs
- 2 - tablespoons grated Parmesan cheese
- 4 - tablespoons chopped parsley for garnish

Instructions:

1. Preheat grill, putting temperature to high. Set broiler rack amidst the range. Line a making ready sheet with thwart.
2. Shower the mushroom tops with olive oil cooking splash on the two facets. Sprinkle with 1/4 teaspoon suit salt, 1/eight teaspoon pepper and 1/four teaspoon garlic powder. Cook five minutes on every aspect, or until simplest delicate.
3. Take off mushrooms from stove. Deplete any fluids. Change range from sear to warmness, putting temperature to 400 levels F.

4. Break an egg into each mushroom. Sprinkle with the cheddar. Prepare 15 mins, until the factor that egg whites are cooked.

5. Sprinkle the eggs with the relaxation of the 1/4 teaspoon salt and 1/eight teaspoon pepper. Trimming with parsley, and serve.

Zucchini Tortilla Ingredients

Ingredients:

- 1 - medium to large Zucchini (6 -7 ounces), cut in large chunks.

- 2-3 - cloves Garlic, minced.

- ½ - Tsp Chipotle pepper powder (or chili powder).

- Dash Sea Salt.

- 2 - Tsp Flax Meal

- 1 - Tbsp Coconut Flour.

- 1 - Egg, beaten.

Breakfast Tostada Ingredients:

- 2 - Zucchini Tortillas.

- 2 - Eggs.

- 2 - Slices of Bacon, nitrate free, cooked and crumbled.

- ½ - Avocado, sliced.

- 1-2 - Tbsp salsa or hot sauce, to taste.

- 1 - Tbsp Cilantro, chopped.

- 1-2 - Tbsp grated cheese.

Instructions:

1. Preheat broiler to 400 F, and line a heating sheet with material paper.
2. Put Zucchini and garlic cloves in sustenance processor or blender, and process till slashed into fine pieces (or could grind zucchini with grater).
3. Place zucchini garlic blend into a cheddar fabric (fine weave towel) or layered paper towel, and press out as much water into sink as you can.
4. Pour blend to a blending dish, and blend every outstanding fixing.
5. Blend until a little thicker (it won' resemble mixture, more like a player).
6. Spoon player onto material paper, utilizing back of spoon to spread into a circle.
7. Try not to make too thin, you shouldn't perceive any paper.
8. Slide back of spoon around external edge of tortilla to make even edges.
9. Heat in stove for 10 to 12 minutes, at that point take out and put another sheet of material paper to finish everything and get the two pieces with tortilla between and flip over and set back onto sheet, at that point gradually peel off material paper over tortilla. now, you could return in broiler to prepare opposite side for 8 to 10 minutes and after that place an officially fricasseed egg over it. Or on the other hand you could cook it any of the accompanying routes underneath:
10. Presently you have a decision of either splitting the egg ideal on the tortilla, on the material paper, and set back in

400 f broiler for 8 minutes or longer depending how you want your egg to be cooked, or you could warm an oiled rotisserie dish on the stove best to medium and place tortilla in sear skillet and break an egg over it. At that point put cover on skillet and broil for a few minutes until the point when egg is cooked how you want.

11. When egg is done, top with cooked bacon disintegrates, avocado, salsa, cilantro, and discretionary cheddar.

Paleo Muffin Recipe

Ingredients:

- 1 - cup any nut butter I have used cashew, peanut, almond, and sunflower seed. My favorite is cashew.

- 2-3 - VERY ripe banana w/ tons of black spots I have also used some prunes to help sweeten in place of the some of the banana

- 2 - eggs I have also tried a chia/flax egg, and while very delicious, the texture is moister and they do not rise as high

- 1 - teaspoon vanilla

- 10 - drops liquid stevia, this amount here greatly depends on personal taste and the sweetness of your bananas.)

- ½ - teaspoon baking soda

- 1 - teaspoon apple cider vinegar

Instructions:

1. Preheat broiler to 400 degrees.
2. Place all fixings into a blender or sustenance processor.
3. Mix until the point that very much blended: player will be sticky.
4. Empty player into a lubed smaller than usual biscuit tins.
5. Heat in a 400-degree stove for 8 minutes or something like that, marginally longer with chia eggs. I am certain you could utilize standard biscuits as well; however, you should expand the cooking time to 12-15 minutes.

Zucchini Blender Bread Recipe

Ingredients:

- 1 - medium zucchini, cut in half and seeds scraped out with a spoon then cut into chunks
- 4 - eggs
- 12 - pitted dates
- ¼ - cup melted butter, ghee or coconut oil
- 1 - teaspoon pure vanilla extract
- ½ - cup coconut flour
- 1 - tablespoon cinnamon
- 1 - teaspoon baking soda
- 1 - tablespoon apple cider vinegar
- ¼ - teaspoon sea salt
- 1/3 - cup chocolate chips, walnuts or any other nuts or seeds

Instructions:

1. Preheat range to 350 degrees F.
2. Include zucchini portions, dates, eggs, spread, and vanilla to a blender and blend till easy.
3. Include the coconut flour, cinnamon, making ready pop, apple juice vinegar and ocean salt and mix by using and by until altogether combined.
4. On the off hazard which you are utilizing any include in's. Include them now and speedy blend.

5. Fill a widespread measured all around lubed (or material covered) portion skillet (I make use of THIS element field) and heat for a hour. Appreciate!

Flourless Pumpkin Pie Muffins

Ingredients:

- ¼ - cup (64 g) almond butter*
- ¾ - cup (180 g) canned pumpkin
- 1 - large egg
- 6 - Tbsp (120 g) honey
- ½ - cup (40 g) rolled oats (GF, if needed)
- 2 - Tbsp (14g) ground flaxseed
- 1 - tsp ground cinnamon
- ½ - tsp ground nutmeg
- ½ - tsp ground cloves
- 1 - tsp vanilla extract
- ½ - tsp baking soda
- ¼ - cup mini chocolate chips, plus more for sprinkling

Instructions:

1. Preheat your broiler to 375F (190C) and installation a biscuit skillet by using splashing nine holes with cooking shower or fixing them with cloth liners. Put aside.
2. Include each one of the fixings other than the chocolate chips to a powerful blender** and mix on excessive till the factor that the oats have separated and the hitter is easy and rich. Mix within the chocolate chips through hand.
3. Disperse the hitter uniformly among the biscuit container cavities, filling each on until the point that it is around 3/4 full.
4. Heat for 18-20 minutes, until the point that the highest points of your biscuits are set and a toothpick embedded into the inside confesses all. Enable the biscuits to cool in the search for gold minutes previously expelling. Store them in a water/air proof compartment for up to 5 days, or stop them for up to 3 months.

Fried Honey Bananas

Ingredients:

- 1 - teaspoon cinnamon
- 1 - tablespoon water
- 1 - tablespoon honey
- 1 - tablespoon coconut oil (olive oil works too!)
- 1 - slightly under-ripened banana

Instructions:

1. Warmth oil in a skillet over medium warm temperature. Cut banana into about ¼ inch thick cuts.
2. Broil bananas for two mins on each aspect, at instances lifting to counteract staying.
3. Whisk together nectar and water. Take off the box from warm and pour nectar and water over bananas.
4. Top with cinnamon.

Cinnamon Roll Recipe with Cream Cheese Icing

Ingredients:

DOUGH:

- ½ - cup warm goat milk
- 1 - package active dry yeast
- 2 - cups cassava flour
- ½ - cup tapioca starch
- 1 - cup boiled sweet potato, mashed
- ¼ - cup coconut sugar
- 4 - tablespoons grass-fed butter
- ½ - teaspoon salt
- 1 - egg

FILLING:

- 1 - cup coconut sugar
- 4 - tablespoons grass-fed butter
- 2 - tablespoons cinnamon
- ¼ - teaspoon cardamom

ICING:

- 4 - ounces raw cream cheese
- 4 - tablespoons grass-fed butter
- ½ - cup coconut sugar
- 1 - tablespoon vanilla extract
- 2 - teaspoons orange zest

Instructions:

1. Preheat range to 350 tiers F. Oil a medium-sized heating dish.
2. In an intensive bowl, combo heat goat drains and yeast. Rest for 10 mins. On the off chance that yeast bunches, start once more.
3. Include batter fixings: cassava, custard, sweet potato, sugar, unfold, egg and salt. Blend till for the maximum part consolidated and after that rubdown with arms into a ball. Cover and relaxation combination for 60 minutes.
4. In a touch bowl, combo filling fixings: sugar, margarine, cinnamon and cardamom. Put aside
5. With cloth on a level floor, flow batter into an expansive rectangular shape about ¼ inch thick.
6. With your hand, unfold the filling equally over the leveled combination.
7. With the assistance of the fabric paper, painstakingly roll the aggregate into itself. Move this as tight as could be allowed.
8. Utilizing a string, tie one bunch around the cinnamon roll. Draw the two sides of the string to intentionally cut the cinnamon roll. Rehash until the factor that each one rolls are reduce.
9. Place every roll onto the lubed making ready dish.
10. Prepare for 15– 20 minutes
11. In a special little bowl, integrate icing fixings: cream cheddar, spread, vanilla and orange pizzazz.
12. Spread what tops off an already right element and serve.

Maple Breakfast Sausage Recipe

Ingredients:

- ½ - cup maple syrup
- 2 - tablespoons ghee
- 1 - pound grass-fed ground beef
- 2 - tablespoons coconut amines

Instructions:

1. In big bowl combine all fixings.
2. Place a griddle over low warmth and include the margarine.
3. Shape meat into frankfurter connections and place in the skillet.
4. Cook with cover on for 15-20 minutes or until cooked through.

Hearty Spinach Beef Frittata Recipe

Ingredients:

- 10 - large eggs, beaten
- 2 - tsp smoked paprika
- ¾ - tsp sea salt
- ½ - tsp black pepper
- 8 to 12 - oz grass-fed ground beef
- 1 - small onion, diced
- 4 oz - mushrooms, sliced (I like shiitake but use what's on hand)
- 10 oz - frozen chopped spinach, defrosted and excess moisture squeezed out
- 1 - large tomato, sliced

Instructions:

1. Preheat the range to 350°F (177°C).
2. In a massive bowl, beat the eggs together with the smoked paprika, salt and pepper. Put aside.
3. In a significant solid press skillet over medium high warmth, sauté the beef till the point that it's cooked thru.
4. Include the onion and mushrooms and sauté until the point whilst they're comfy and marginally sensitive.
5. Include the defrosted and depleted spinach. Blend to join.

6. Empty the egg combo into the skillet. Kill the warm temperature and blend the fixings to sign up for.
7. Lay the tomato cuts to complete the entirety.
8. Heat for round 20 minutes or until the factor whilst the eggs are set and now not runny.
9. Serve mainly from the skillet or reduce and keep for final.

Oatmeal Cottage Cheese Banana Pancakes

Ingredients:

- ½ - cup gluten-free old-fashioned rolled oats
- ½ - medium banana
- ½ - teaspoon vanilla extract
- 1 - teaspoon baking powder
- ½ - teaspoon cinnamon
- 2 - large egg whites (or 1 egg)
- ¼ - cup fat free (or low-fat) cottage cheese
- 1-2 - tablespoons unsweetened vanilla almond milk
- Fresh berries, chocolate chips, peanut butter

Instructions:

1. Place all fixings in a blender and blend till the factor when totally easy, round 30 seconds.
2. Softly coat an expansive nonstick skillet or frying pan with margarine or cooking shower and heat over medium low warm temperature. Drop participant by way of 1/4 field onto skillet. Include wanted fixings, as an instance, chocolate chips or blueberries. Cook until the point whilst bubbles display up to finish everything. Flip desserts and cook dinner until outstanding darkish colored on underside. Wipe skillet clean and rehash with moreover cooking splash and ultimate hitter. Makes three-four flapjacks.

Paleo Breakfast Casserole

Ingredients:

- 12 - eggs

- 1 - large sweet potato

- ½ - cup spinach

- Salt and pepper, to taste

- Coconut oil, for coating

- ½ - lb. ground meat,

  turkey or beef

Instructions:

1. Preheat the range to 350 F. Coat a nine x 9 warming plate with coconut oil.
2. Cook floor meat in a skillet with coconut oil, until burned. Season nicely at some point of cooking.
3. Cut the sweet potato into cuts round 1/4 inch thick. Layer the cuts on the warming plate.
4. Top the sweet potatoes with the floor meat, and unrefined spinach.
5. Whisk 12 eggs well. Season with salt and pepper to taste. Pour to cover the blend totally.
6. Heat in the stove for 40-45 minutes, or until the point that sweet potatoes have diminished and eggs are cooked through.

Breakfast Pizza

Ingredients:

- 1 - cup tapioca flour
- One egg
- 1 - tbsp olive oil
- 1 - tbsp water
- add any spices you love

Instructions:

1. Preheat broiler to 375.
2. Join fixings until the point that a wet batter shapes, this does not feel like your run of the mill mixture.
3. Spread it out equally and daintily.

Top with:

Ingredients:

Just blend basil, garlic, parsley, olive oil and pine nuts until smooth. homemade or bought pesto

- ✓ slices of tomato
- ✓ two eggs
- ✓ Romano cheese. optional

Kale Salad with Mushroom Omelet Recipe

Ingredients:

FOR THE SALAD

- 1 - tablespoon miso paste (or 1 teaspoon soy sauce)

- 4 - eggs

- 1 - tablespoon olive oil

- 2 - cups chopped mushrooms of your choice

- 8 - big handfuls chopped kale, tough stems discarded

- ½ - teaspoon kosher salt

- 1/3 - cup unsalted chopped raw pecans or walnuts

- 3 - ounces grated Pecorino Romano cheese

FOR THE LEMON-CHILE VINAIGRETTE

- 1 - clove garlic, finely minced

- ½ - teaspoon kosher salt

- 1/3 - cup freshly squeezed lemon juice

- 1 - teaspoon Chile oil or Chile sauce (optional)

- 2 - tablespoons extra virgin olive oil

- 2 - teaspoons Dijon mustard

- 2 - teaspoons honey

- freshly ground black pepper

Instructions:

1. Make the serving of mixed greens dressing by consolidating the vinaigrette fixings in a jug with a tight-fitting top (like a bricklayer container) and shake well to join. Taste and include more salt as required.
2. Whisk the miso glue with the eggs. Warmth a griddle over medium-high warmth and whirl in the olive oil. Include the mushrooms and sauté for 2 minutes, or until the point that mushrooms relaxed. Include the egg and turn the warmth to medium. Let cook for 2 minutes. Cover and let cook for an extra 1-2 minutes or until the point that eggs are set.
3. While eggs are cooking, put the kale in an extensive bowl. Sprinkle with salt. Utilizing rubbing movement, rub the kale leaves together to separate and diminish the kale.
4. At the point when prepared to serve, cut omelet in strips. Hurl kale with a portion of the dressing (I utilized around 1/4 measure of the dressing), hacked nuts and Pecorino Romano cheddar. Present with omelet

Paleo Breakfast Porridge Recipe

Ingredients:

- 2 - ripe bananas (or one large, very ripe, plantain), mashed
- 2 - cups coconut milk (or 1 can plus extra water)
- ¾ - cup almond meal
- ¼ - cup flax meal
- 1 - teaspoon cinnamon
- ½ - teaspoon ginger
- 1/8 - teaspoon ground cloves
- 1/8 - teaspoon ground nutmeg
- 1/8 teaspoon Celtic sea salt
- maple syrup or raw honey (optional)
- toppings like berries, unsweetened coconut flakes, nuts, seeds, etc.... (optional)
- 2 - ripe bananas (or one large, very ripe, plantain), mashed
- 2 - cups coconut milk (or 1 can plus extra water)

Instructions:

1. Consolidate all fixings in a medium pan and warmth to a moderate stew, blending, until thick and bubbly.
2. The consistency will change contingent upon the kind of coconut drain you utilize. (I as a rule utilize "light" coconut drain) The blend will appear to be thin at first however thicken up rapidly. It will keep on thickening

after it is served so you may need to include additional water or coconut drain.

Paleo Breakfast Porridge

3. I seek you appreciate this formula after paleo breakfast porridge. For more paleo breakfast formulas and thoughts check here.
4. Instead of depending on oat substitutes on a more extended term premise, it is best to utilize this as a more transitional formula. It is intended to enable you to make the move to less dependence on oats and gives some regularly required assortment

Paleo Cinnamon Raisin Bagels

Ingredients:

- 1/3 - cup coconut flour sifted

- 1 ½ - Tbsp golden flax meal

- ½ - tsp baking soda or can use 1 tsp baking powder.

- 2 - tsp cinnamon.

- A dash sea salt

- 3 - eggs beaten.

- 1/3 - cup unsweetened coconut or almond milk.

- 2 ½ - tbsp butter melted, or coconut oil or ghee, melted, where to buy coconut oil

- 1 - tsp apple cider vinegar.

- 1 - tbsp organic honey or for low carb version use 1 tsp liquid stevia., paleo

- 1 - tsp organic GF vanilla extract.

- 1/3 - cup golden or dark unsculptured raisins, or for lowest carb, omit raisins and make plain bagels * optional, can omit raisins for making plain bagels.

- Kitchen tools:

- 1 - bagel donut mold pan where to buy bagel pan [

- 2 - large mixing bowls

Instructions:

1. Start Oven to 350 F, and oil or oil a bagel or donut dish (about six donut skillet)
2. In a vast bowl Add: 1/3 field sifted coconut flour, 1 ½ tbsp superb flax dinner, half tsp warming pop or 1 tsp influencing prepared to powder, 2 tsp cinnamon (non-necessary), 1/8 tsp sea salt. Include all completely.
3. In another blending, dish consolidates 3 eggs, 1/3 glass coconut or almond drain, 2 ½ tbsp spread or coconut oil (liquefied), 1 tsp apple juice vinegar, 1 tbsp nectar or low carb choice 1 tsp stevia, 1 tsp vanilla concentrate. Combine altogether.
4. Add wet fixings to the dry (coconut flour blend). Combine completely.
5. Include discretionary raisins or stop dried (or crisp) blueberries to blend and mix.
6. Spoon player into bagel or doughnut container and spread around with the back of a spoon. Utilize a sodden material or paper towel to wipe off bagel focus.
7. Heat at 350 F for17 to 20 minutes, check at 17 minutes.
8. Take off from the stove, and let bagels cool. Utilize a margarine cut amongst bagel and skillet edges, and slide around to release bagels.
9. Can be turned up on the side and cut into equal parts. Could skillet toast in lubed or buttered sear container on the two sides till caramelized. Could likewise utilize a toaster stove or stove grill to toast. *Don't utilize a standard toaster as they may fall apart*
10. Present with fixing of decision: spread, sunflower margarine, almond spread, coconut spread, nectar, creamy cheddar and so on....
11. Refrigerate or stop unused parts.

Pancake Buns

Ingredients:

- 2 -organic cage-free eggs
- ¾ - cup of unsweetened vanilla almond milk
- 2 - tablespoons canned coconut milk, full fat (refrigerated over the night)
- 1 - tablespoon coconut nectar
- 1 - tablespoon pure maple syrup, grade B
- 1 - tablespoon coconut oil (melted)
- 1 - tablespoon carbonated water (makes the pancakes fluffy!)
- 1 & ½ - teaspoon vanilla
- 1 & ¾ - cup sifted blanched almond flour
- 1 - teaspoon of baking powder
- ½ - teaspoon sea salt
- 1/8 - teaspoon cinnamon

Instructions:

1. Warmth a medium estimated dish or skillet on low warmth while you set up the hotcake player.
2. Put the eggs in a nourishment processor or blender and blend. At that point include the wet fixings: almond drain, coconut drain, coconut nectar, maple syrup, coconut oil, carbonated water, vanilla concentrate and

blend once more. Presently include the staying dry fixings: almond flour, preparing powder, ocean salt, and cinnamon. Blend until joined. The player will have a fluid consistency somewhat more slender than customary hotcake hitter, don't fuss!

3. Coat the skillet with your decision of against stick covering or splash, I utilized coconut oil. Turn the stove up to medium warmth and empty the measure of player into the dish as indicated by your coveted flapjack estimate. These infants will have little gaps that begin to rise on top when the base is prepared simply like normal flapjacks do, so you'll know when to flip them. Ensure the base is totally done, else they may disintegrate because of their sensitive consistency. They are Paleo all things considered, there is no gluten to "stick" them together. I recommend utilizing an Egg/Pancake Ring which function admirably to shape and cook your hotcakes. Simply fill one midway and let the hotcake cook. When it begins to rise at the best softly lift the ring, if any player begins to leak out the base, let it cook longer. At that point utilize a spatula to flip it over once it's prepared. After you're finished cooking the hotcake buns, put aside and begin making your egg patty, hotdog as well as bacon.

Egg Patty

Ingredients:

- 2 - organic cage-free eggs
- splash of water
- pinch of sea salt
- pinch of ground pepper

Instructions:

I tossed everything in a bowl and beat with a hand blender to make the eggs super cushioned. Coat the skillet with your decision of hostile to stick covering or shower, once more, I utilized coconut oil. Turn the stove up to medium warmth and cook the egg like you would an omelet, at that point overlay to a size that will fit on your flapjack bun. Or on the other hand utilize the Egg Ring specified previously. Duh.

Paleo and Keto Egg Muffin Recipe

Ingredients:

- 8oz- Pork Breakfast Sausage

- 1 - Tbl Extra Virgin Olive Oil

- ½ - Sweet Onion (thinly sliced)

- ¾ - Cup Red Bell Peppers (chopped or thinly sliced, any color)

- 1 ½ - Cups Fresh Spinach (packed)

- 1 - tsp Fresh Oregano (chopped or ½ t. dry oregano)

- 9 - Eggs

- Ground Pepper

- ¾ - tsp Real Salt

- ¼ - Cup Coconut Milk

Instructions:

- Preheat stove to 350 degrees. Oil a biscuit tin.
- Place the ground hotdog in a sauté dish and warmth on medium high. Separate the pork into disintegrates with a spatula as it cooks.
- At the point when the pork is mostly cooked, include 1 T. of olive oil, onions, peppers, and oregano to the dish. Sauté until the point that the onion is translucent. Add the spinach to the dish and cover with a top. Cook for 30 seconds, evacuate the cover and hurl the fixings.

Spinach ought to be shriveled yet at the same time splendid green. Take off from warm.

- Place the eggs in an extensive blending dish alongside the pepper, salt, and drain. Whisk together until the point that eggs are well beaten.
- Add the wiener and vegetables to the egg blend and blend in until the point when very much conveyed.
- Partition the mix between the lubed scone tins (12 signify), guaranteeing that each tin has a to some degree level with extent of eggs/fillings.
- Get ready in preheated oven for 18-20 minutes. Cool for two or three minutes and Take out from tins, unwinding the edges first with a sharp edge.

Peach Cobbler Oatmeal

Ingredients:

- 3 ½ - cups water
- pinch of salt
- 2 ½ - cups rolled oats
- 2 ¼ - tsp. cinnamon
- pinch of nutmeg
- 2 - large peaches, chopped
- 3-4 - tablespoons light brown sugar
- ¼ - cup chopped pecans for garnish; if desired

Instructions:

1. In a huge pot over medium warmth, include water and salt. Heat to the point of boiling. Include oats, cinnamon and nutmeg and mix to join.
2. Cook for 4 minutes, or until the point that oats thicken. Include peaches and dark colored sugar and cook one extra moment. Serve promptly and embellish with pecans, if wanted.

Pumpkin Pie Oatmeal Recipe

Ingredients:

- 2 - cups coconut milk
- ⅔ - cup steel cut oats
- ½ - cup pumpkin puree
- ½ - tablespoon chia seeds
- ½ - teaspoon vanilla extract
- pinch of sea salt
- ½ - teaspoon cinnamon
- ¼ - teaspoon ginger
- ⅛ - teaspoon nutmeg

Instructions:

1. In a medium estimated pot, pour in coconut drain and convey to a low bubble.
2. Include oats and swing to down to stew.
3. Include pumpkin puree and chia seeds and keep stewing 5-7 minutes.
4. Include vanilla, salt, cinnamon, ginger and nutmeg.
5. Stew for extra 5-7 minutes or until the point that oats are cooked through.

Gluten-Free Vegan
Raspberry Almond Squares

Ingredients:

- 1 - tbsp ground flax seeds

- 3 - tbsp very warm water

- 2 ½ - cups almonds

- ⅓ - cup liquid sweetener of your choice

- ⅓ - cup coconut oil, melted or very soft

- 1 - tsp pure vanilla extract

- ¼ - tsp salt

- 1 - cup raspberry jam of your choice

- ½ - cup sliced almonds

Instructions:

1. Preheat stove to 350F. Line a 8×8 preparing dish (or anything of a comparable size) with some material paper.
2. Influence a flax to egg by blending the ground flax in warm water in a little glass. Blend and put aside to gel for a couple of minutes.
3. Process almonds in a sustenance processor until ground just somewhat coarser than almond flour. Include your sweetener, coconut oil, vanilla, salt, and flax egg, and process until the point when everything is joined.

4. Empty the blend into the readied heating dish and prepare for 22 minutes until the point that the base turns out to be somewhat brilliant and springs back when contacted softly.
5. Take off the preparing dish from the stove (keep broiler running however). Spread raspberry stick equally finished the best. Sprinkle cut almonds equally over the stick. Return back to stove and heat for an extra 15 minutes until the point when the almonds start to get somewhat brilliant.
6. Take off from stove and cool on a rack. When cool, cut into squares and appreciate. I like these warm actually, yet my significant other preferences chilled treats better, so in case you're that sort of individual then simply refrigerate for an hour or two to chill.

Paleo Raspberry Pop Tarts

Ingredients:
DOUGH

- ¼ - cup water

- ¼ - cup ghee

- ¼ - cup B grade maple syrup

- 1 - teaspoon pure vanilla extract

- ¼ - teaspoon sea salt

- ½ - cup tapioca flour

- 1 - medium ripe banana mashed

- ½ cup coconut flour

RASPBERRY FILLING

- 1 ½ - cup fresh raspberries

- ¼ - cup water

- ½ - teaspoon pure vanilla extract

- ¼ - teaspoon sea salt

- 2 - Tablespoon B grade maple syrup

Instructions:

1. For the aggregate: In a medium sauce dish, encompass the water, ghee, maple syrup, vanilla and ocean salt and heat to the point of boiling. Expel from the stove top.
2. Include the custard flour and blend with a spoon till consolidated.
3. At that factor include the squashed banana and coconut flour and blend until the factor if you have a batter.
4. Put apart.

For the raspberry filling:

5. In a medium sauce dish include the raspberries, water, vanilla, salt and maple syrup and prepare dinner on medium warm temperature for 35 - 45 minutes. It should decrease significantly.
6. Take the batter and flow it out between two sheets of material paper until the factor that the aggregate is 1/4". Cut into rectangular shapes and spoon 2 tbsps. of raspberry filling onto one square shape and cover with any other rectangular form. You should have 12 square shapes - around 2" - three". You may have extra mixture which goes outstanding for thumbprints.
7. Prepare on a bit of material paper inside the broiler for 25 mins at 350 ranges. Appreciate!

Raw Apple-Cinnamon & Chia Breakfast Bowl

Ingredients:

- 3 - honey crisp apples, peeled and cored, divided
- 4-5 - medjool dates, pitted
- ½ - teaspoon ground cinnamon
- pinch nutmeg
- 2 - tablespoons chia seeds
- Toppings
- raw walnuts
- raisins
- dried cranberries
- hemp seeds

Instructions:

1. Nicely diced one of the Honeycrisp apples and add to an impermeable holder.
2. Take two of the Honeycrisp apples and cut them into extensive pieces. Add the apple pieces to a sustenance processor alongside the dates, cinnamon, and nutmeg. Heartbeat the blend a few times and afterward let it process for 2-3 minutes, ceasing sometimes to rub the blend down the sides. Empty the apple-date blend into the holder with the diced apple and mix in the chia seeds.
3. Put it in Refrigerate for 1 hour or medium-term.
4. Gap the apple blend between two bowls and best with crude walnuts, raisins, cranberries, and hemp seeds.
5. Serve and appreciate.
6. Refrigerate remains.

Sage Chicken Breakfast Patties Recipe

Ingredients:

- ¼ - teaspoon black pepper
- ¼ - teaspoon sea salt
- 1 - teaspoon ground sage
- ½ - teaspoon onion powder
- ¼ - teaspoon garlic powder
- ¼ - teaspoon Basil
- 1 - tablespoon Parsley
- 1 - large apple, peeled and diced
- 1 - pound organic ground chicken

Instructions:

1. Consolidate every one of the fixings in bowl and blend. Shape blend into singular patties.
2. Warmth an expansive skillet with coconut oil over medium high warmth. Include chicken patties and cook for around 6-8 minutes on each side.

Shakshuka

Ingredients:

- 1 - yellow onion, sliced
- 1 - cup fresh organic spinach
- 1 - red bell pepper, sliced
- 1 - can organic diced tomatoes
- 1 - tbsp extra-virgin olive oil
- 2 - gluten-free chicken sausages (I use spicy), sliced down the middle or cut into pieces (Optional)
- 1 - tsp chili powder
- ½ - tsp cumin
- ¼ - tsp Himalayan sea salt
- ¼ - tsp cayenne pepper, more as desired Optional
- ¼ - tsp turmeric Optional
- 4 - fresh organic, pasture-raised eggs
- Chopped parsley, for garnish

Instructions:

1. Warmth oil in a skillet
2. Include cut onions and red ringer pepper, sauté for 5 minutes until translucent
3. Include wiener and spinach, let frankfurter cook and spinach shrivel

4.   Include diced tomatoes, bean stew powder, ocean salt, cumin, and cayenne; blend to mix very well
5.   Tenderly spread a zone and split an egg in, proceed with outstanding eggs
6.   Let cook until the point when egg whites are hazy
7.   For speedier cooking, cover your skillet
8.   Trimming with parsley, extra cayenne pepper, and crisply split dark pepper

3-Ingredient Banana Pudding Recipe

Ingredients:

- 1 - ripe banana peeled
- ¼ - cup full-fat coconut milk
- 2 - tbsp chia seeds

Instructions:

1. In a sustenance processor or blender, consolidate the banana and coconut drain. Process until easy.
2. Include the chia seeds and heartbeat a couple of instances to blend uniformly.
3. Fill a compartment and sit back for a hour to allow the chia seeds stout up a bit. (Or however if you're just like me, spoil it proper since you will opt for not to pause. The seeds could be crunchy, however.)

Turkey Sausage, Broccoli & Tomato Crestless Quiche

Ingredients:

- 8oz -1 ¼ - cups sliced cooked breakfast turkey sausage links, or cooked, crumbled sausage
- 1 - medium or about 1 cup chopped tomato
- 1 - cup chopped broccoli, steamed or frozen and thawed
- 6 - eggs
- ½ - cup milk
- ½ - teaspoon kosher salt
- ½ - teaspoon freshly ground black pepper
- ½ - teaspoon dry mustard
- 1 - cup shredded cheddar cheese

Instructions:

1. Preheat the stove to 400°F, and coat a 9-inch glass pie plate with oil or cooking shower.
2. Layer wiener, tomato, broccoli in arranged pie plate, and best with the destroyed cheddar.
3. Whisk together the eggs, drain, salt, pepper, and dry mustard, and pour over the meat and cheddar in the pie plate.
4. Prepare for 35-40 minutes, or until the point that egg is cooked through and top is caramelized.

Turmeric Eggs Recipe

Ingredients:

- 4 - eggs
- 2 - ounces raw cheese, shredded
- 3 - tablespoons ghee
- ½ - cup red onions, chopped
- 8 - green onions, chopped
- 1 - cup yellow peppers, chopped
- 6 - cloves of garlic, minced
- 1 - tablespoon thyme
- 1 - tablespoon oregano
- 1 - tablespoon basil
- 2 - tablespoons turmeric

Instructions:

1. Sauté onions, green onions and garlic in container with ghee over medium-low warmth for 10 minutes.
2. Include eggs, cheddar and herbs.
3. Cook for 10 minutes, mixing constantly and include turmeric.

Vanilla Chia Pudding Recipe

Ingredients:

- ¾ - cup almond milk, unsweetened
- 1 - tbsp maple syrup or honey*
- 1 - tsp pure vanilla extract
- 3 - tbsp chia seeds
- (optional) Nuts, berries, fruit, coconut flakes for topping

Instructions:

1. In any glass with a decent seal pinnacle, encompass fixings in the accompanying request: drain, maple syrup, vanilla and chia seeds. In the occasion which you might need to consist of fixings towards the beginning of the day, utilize more jugs, normally make use of littler bins (imagined).
2. Mix well with a spoon or fork, allow sit for 1 second and blend yet again. This will avoid bumps. At that factor refrigerate medium-term.
3. At the factor whilst organized to eat, combo nicely and best with most cherished garnishes: nuts, berries, organic product, coconut drops and so on.

Veggie Quiche Cups To-Go

Ingredients:

- 7 - eggs or 1 ¾ c. egg substitute
- ¾ c - shredded cheddar cheese
- ¼ c - finely diced red bell pepper
- ¼ c - finely diced mushrooms
- ¼ c - finely diced onion
- 1 (10 oz.) - package frozen
- chopped spinach, thawed and
  well-drained

Instructions:

1. Line 12 biscuit glasses with thwart heating containers; shower with non-stick cooking splash.
2. Add all fixings in a bowl and blend well.
3. Partition the blend equitably between the biscuit mugs. Heat at 350 degrees for 20-25 minutes, until the point that set and a blade embedded in the inside tells the truth.
4. Store refrigerated. Expel from thwart liners and warm in the microwave when you're prepared to eat them.

2 Minute Paleo Porridge

Ingredients:

- 1 - very ripe banana
- 1/3 - cup of shredded coconut
- 2 - Tablespoons of cashew butter

TOPPINGS:

- Nuts
- Dried fruit
- fresh berries
- Cinnamon
- Coconut Butter

Instructions:

1. Crush the banana together with the destroyed coconut and cashew margarine.
2. I utilized a fork to crush everything together. Top with crisp berries or slashed nuts.

Sheet Pan Classic Breakfast

Ingredients:

- 2 - large yellow potatoes, cleaned and diced to ½
- 1 - medium onion, small dice
- 1 - red or green bell pepper, small dice
- 1 - teaspoon avocado oil
- ½ - teaspoon garlic powder
- ½ - teaspoon chili powder
- ½ - teaspoon dried parsley
- 6 - pieces nitrate-free bacon
- 4 - pasture-raised eggs, more as desired
- Salt and fresh ground pepper, to taste

Instructions:

1. Pre-warm stove to 400ºF and line a rimmed preparing sheet with material paper.
2. In an expansive bowl join diced potato, chime pepper, onion, avocado oil, and flavors. Hurl to consolidate and pour onto a rimmed preparing sheet.
3. Place in broiler and heat for 20 minutes.
4. Take out container and move vegetable blend to the other side of the skillet. Add bacon in strips to the opposite side and come back to broiler for 12 minutes.
5. Take off from stove and move bacon to the side. Move the hash dark colored blend around with abundance bacon fat to get the potatoes decent and fresh. Move

potatoes back to the side and make four little divots in potatoes to break the eggs. Break eggs in the divots and come back to broiler to prepare for 8-10 minutes. Heat until the point that eggs are cooked for wanted surface. 8 minutes are delicate runny yellow yolks or 10 minutes for all the more completely heated eggs.

6. Plate the hash tans and eggs on to a plate and quickly deplete the bacon of overabundance fat on paper towel before plating and serving. Salt and pepper to taste (yet taste first as the bacon adds salt to the dish.

Maple Pecan Grain-Free Granola

Ingredients:

- 1 - cup pecans or walnuts

- ¾ - cup slivered almonds

- ¼ - cup shredded coconut

- ¼ - cup pumpkin seeds

- 3 - tbsp ground chia seeds

- 1 - tsp cinnamon non-irradiated

- ¼ - tsp sea salt

- 2 - tbsp maple syrup

- 1 - tbsp coconut oil

- ¼ - cup raisins

Instructions:

1. Join all fixings apart from the raisins in a bowl and mix well to fuse the maple syrup and chia seeds with exchange fixings. Ensure you dissolve the coconut oil before you mixt it with exchange fixings.
2. Spread the combination on a heating sheet fixed with fabric paper. Prepare at 300° to 325° (contingent upon your broiler warm, mine has an inclination to get surprisingly hot, so I completed 300°) and heat, mixing part of the way through, for round 10-15 mins or until the point while the granola is fresh and incredible darkish colored, remember in order now not to eat.
3. Take off granola from the stove and permit cool, at that factor encompass the raisins. The raisins will be predisposed to get too difficult at the off danger that you warmth them within the broiler, so I like to position drizzle with complete fat coconut drain
4. For guidelines on the maximum talented approach to make cooked grew quinoa, visit me submit Ho2. When quinoa is completed cooking, yet on the equal time heat include coconut oil. It will liquefy as your combination it round, at that factor include coconut sugar.
5. Include berries of your choice. I applied new natural blueberries and cleaved strawberries.
6. Shower coconut drain over the berries. Appreciate!

Grain-Free Granola

Ingredients:

- 8 - cups mixed nuts
- 4 - large egg whites (1/2 cup)
- 4 - tablespoons maple syrup (1/4 cup) or to taste
- 2 - tablespoons vanilla extract
- 4 - teaspoons cinnamon
- 1 - teaspoon ginger
- 1 - teaspoon allspice
- 2-4 - tablespoons coconut oil or butter

Instructions:

1. Whisk or beat egg whites with the maple syrup, vanilla extract, and spices in a big bowl till blended.
2. Cut up nuts to most well-known length, a meals processor will make this clean, and mix into the egg aggregate.
3. Butter or oil the insert of a sluggish cooker and pour in the nut mixture.
4. Turn on the ease back cooker to high and cook granola, blending each 15-20 minutes, until the point when the covering dries (around 2-3 hours).
5. Permit to cool before putting away in a hermetically sealed holder. Any dried natural product or extra blend ins can be included after it cools.

Avocado Sweet Potato Toast with Poached Egg

Ingredients:

- 1 - sweet potato
- 4 - Egg's
- 1 - avocado
- Sea salt
- Red pepper flakes
- Micro greens for garnish

Instructions:

1. Heat the stove to 400°F. Clean the sweet potato and trim off pointy closes. On a cutting board, lay sweet potato on its side and cut into ¼ inch. Place the sweet potato cuts on a baking pan. Bake for 15 minutes, till the point that the sweet potatoes are really soft.
2. While the sweet potato is warming, scoop out the substance of the avocado into a bowl. Season with a press of sea salt and dull pepper. Pound with a fork until smooth and rich. Set aside.
3. Poach your eggs: Bring a little pan of water to a bubble, and after that decrease it to a stew. Break one egg at any given moment into a little serving dish or estimating container so you don't need to split it specifically into the spewing water. Gradually mix the water in a roundabout movement as you tenderly slide the egg

into the water, cooking for 3– 4 minutes. Take out the egg with a strainer scoop and place on a plate secured with a paper towel.

4. At the point when sweet potato toasts are prepared, take off from the stove and place each cut on a serving plate. Spread the pounded avocado over the sweet potato toast and best with poached eggs. Season with ocean salt and red pepper drops and topping best with miniaturized scale greens.

Mushroom Risotto with Cauliflower Rice

Ingredients:

- 1 - large head cauliflower, cut into florets

- 1T - coconut oil

- 1 - large yellow onion, diced

- 2 - large garlic cloves, minced

- ¾ - lb. mushrooms, thinly sliced

- ½ - cup beef stock

- Fresh parsley, chopped

- Salt and pepper, to taste

Instructions:

1. Cut the cauliflower into little florets, at that point wash and dry them with paper towels.
2. Process the cauliflower florets in little bunches in a nourishment processor or blender until the point that you get a rice-like surface.
3. Warmth coconut oil in a vast skillet over medium warmth and sauté the onions until the point when they are delicate and caramelized (around 5 minutes). Include the garlic and mix until the point that it is fragrant. Include the mushrooms and sauté until the point when mushrooms are darker on the two sides.
4. Include the cauliflower rice and hamburger stock and convey warm down to low. Permit the cauliflower rice to retain the meat stock until the point when it is delicate yet not soft (around 10 minutes).
5. Add salt and pepper to taste. Trimming with hacked new parsley before isolating it into dishes and serving.

Thai Red Curry Chicken

Ingredients:

- ½ - teaspoon salt

- ¼ - teaspoon pepper

- sriracha to taste (optional)

- Garnish

- lime zest to taste

- fresh basil

- fresh cilantro

- fresh lime juice

- 1 - small zucchini, sliced

- 1 - bay leaf

- 1 ½ - tablespoons olive oil or coconut oil

- 1 - pound chicken breasts sliced into ¼" slices then 2" pieces

- ½ - large onion, chopped

- 2 - tablespoons red curry paste

- 1 - red bell pepper, thinly sliced then chopped into 2" pieces

- 1 - orange bell pepper thinly sliced then chopped into 2" pieces

- 2 - teaspoons freshly grated ginger

- 4 - garlic cloves, minced

- 13.5oz. can quality coconut milk

- 1 - tablespoon cornstarch

- 1 - tablespoon Asian/Thai Sweet Chili Sauce

- 2 - tablespoons less sodium soy sauce

- 2 - tablespoon fish sauce

- 2 - tablespoons lime juice

- 1 - tablespoon brown sugar

- 1 - teaspoon dried basil

Instructions:

1. Warmth oil over medium-high warmth in a big pot. Add all; chicken, onion and pink curry glue and prepare dinner simply till the point while the chicken is no pinker. Add all; ringer peppers, zucchini, ginger and garlic and sauté 1 minute.
2. Include 1/2 of the coconut drain. Blend final coconut drain with 1 tablespoon cornstarch and upload to skillet alongside each single extremely good fixing (anticipate Garnishes).
3. Warmth to the point of bubbling, at that factor reduce to a stew for 5 mins or until the point that the sauce thickens and the greens increase needed shimmering delicacy. In the occasion which you may require a more noteworthy slim sauce, thin with water (I don't attempt this). Discard bay leaf.
4. Finishing with more optional new basil, cilantro, lime spirit, lime juice and Sriracha to taste. Give rice.

Roasted Cauliflower Steaks AND Lemon Dill Tahini Sauce

Ingredients:

For the cauliflower:

- large head of organic cauliflower
- 1 tablespoon 100% pure avocado oil

For the seasoning:

- 1 - tablespoon organic dried dill
- ½ - teaspoon organic ground cumin
- ¼ - teaspoon organic ground garlic powder
- ¼ - teaspoon organic ground black pepper
- ¼ - teaspoon Himalayan pink salt

For the tahini sauce:

- 2 - tablespoons organic lemon juice
- 2 - tablespoons organic tahini
- ¼ - teaspoon organic dried dill
- ¼ - teaspoon organic ground black pepper
- 1/8 - ¼ - teaspoon Himalayan pink salt

Instructions:

1. Preheat broiler to 350 stages.
2. Cauliflower:
3. area the cauliflower on a cutting board with the stem down and the crown confronting upward. exactly reduce the cauliflower from the best (crown) to the stem, taking consideration to keep the cuts unblemished. You ought to get no less than four thick cuts.
4. Place the cauliflower cuts on a heating container fixed with material paper.
5. Rub the avocado oil on the two sides of the cauliflower cuts. Put aside.
6. Flavoring:
7. Include every one of the elements for the flavoring to a little bowl and blend so every one of the fixings are very much consolidated. Alter the seasonings to your inclination.
8. Sprinkle the flavoring on the two sides of every cauliflower cut.
9. Cooking the cauliflower:
10. Place the preparing dish in the broiler at 350 degrees and meal for around a hour, or until the point when the outside edges of the cauliflower are brilliant and within the cauliflower is delicate.
11. Tahini sauce:
12. While the cauliflower is simmering, include every one of the elements for the sauce to a little bowl and whisk together until the point when very much joined. Modify the seasonings to your inclination.
13. Once the cauliflower is done, exchange the cuts to your serving dishes and shower with the tahini sauce.

Basil and Artichoke Shirataki Fettuccine Pasta

Ingredients:

- 2 - packs Shirataki Fettuccine Pasta (Miracle Noodles)

For the sauce:

- ¼ - cups organic pine nuts
- ¾ - cup homemade almond milk
- 2 - tablespoons organic lemon juice (freshly squeezed)
- 2 - tablespoons nutritional yeast
- 2 - cloves organic garlic (freshly crushed)
- 1 - tablespoon organic extra-virgin olive oil
- ½ - teaspoon Himalayan pink salt
- ½ - teaspoon organic ground black pepper

For the add-ins:

- 8 - leaves fresh organic basil (chopped)
- 1 - can artichoke hearts (chopped), (14 ounce can)

Instructions:

1. Set up the supernatural occurrence noodles:
2. Set up the Miracle Noodles as per the bundle headings. Put aside.
3. Set up the include ins:
4. Cleave the basil into long strips and slash the artichokes into little pieces. Put aside.
5. Set up the sauce:

6. Include all elements for the sauce to a Vitamix and mix until it's velvety and smooth. Alter the seasonings to your inclination.
7. Get together:
8. Set the readied noodles, add-ins and sauce to a medium-sized blending dish and delicately hurl until the point that everything is equally appropriated.
9. Place to your serving dishes.
10. Discretionary: Garnish with additional slashed basil.

Gluten-Free Vegan Carrot "Hot Dog"

Ingredients:

- 4 - organic carrots (large and thick)

For the seasoning:

- 1 - teaspoon organic garlic powder

- 1 - teaspoon non-GMO smoked paprika

- 1 - teaspoon Himalayan pink salt

- 1 – teaspoon organic ground black pepper*

Instructions:

1. Set the oven heat to 425 degrees.
   Carrots:
2. Cut the closures off the carrots and chop them down to fit the span of your wiener buns. Mesh the outside skin off the carrots so they are smooth.
3. Fill a cooking pot with sifted/cleansed water and heat to the point of boiling.
4. Place the carrots in the cooking pot and bubble for 20 minutes.
5. Deplete and promptly include the seasonings in the following stage.
   Seasoning:
6. You'll need to include the flavoring quickly in the wake of expelling the carrots from the bubbling water, so they are as yet wet and the seasonings will adhere to the carrots.
7. Choice 1: If your flavoring compartments have the best that you can sprinkle out the seasonings, it's best to sprinkle each flavoring over the carrots in the sum to your inclination. Simply hold the carrot and turn it around as you sprinkle ensuring it's secured the distance around.
8. Alternative 2: If your flavoring compartments don't have the best that you can sprinkle out the seasonings, include every one of the seasonings into a bowl sufficiently extensive to fit the carrots, at that point delicately hurl every carrot in the seasonings until it's secured the distance around.
   Finish cooking the carrots:
9. Place the prepared carrots on a heating dish fixed with material paper and heat at 425 minutes for 10-20 minutes, or until the point when they are sufficiently delicate to your inclination.
10. Remove the carrots from the stove and present with sans gluten frank buns with your most loved fixings like natural ketchup, natural mustard, red onions, and so forth.

Cilantro Pesto Sweet Potato Salad

Ingredients:

For the sweet potatoes:

- 2 - cups organic cubed sweet potatoes
- 1-2 - pinches Himalayan pink salt
- 1-2 - pinches organic ground black pepper

For the cilantro pesto:

- 2 - cups organic fresh cilantro
- ½ - cup organic pine nuts
- ½ - cup organic extra-virgin olive oil
- 1/3 - cup nutritional yeast
- 3 - cloves organic garlic
- 3 - tablespoons organic apple cider vinegar
- ½ - teaspoon Himalayan pink salt
- ½ - teaspoon organic ground black pepper

Instructions:

1. Preheat stove to 350 degrees.
2. Peel and cut sweet potatoes into little 3D squares. You will require 2 mugs for this formula.

3. Place the sweet potato 3D squares on a heating skillet fixed with material paper.
4. Sprinkle 1-2 squeezes of Himalayan pink salt and natural ground pepper equally finished the sweet potato solid shapes.
5. Prepare in the broiler at 350 degrees for roughly 30-35 minutes, or until the point that they are delicate.
6. While the sweet potatoes are heating, include all fixings (fluids first) to a Vitamix and mix until it's very much consolidated, utilizing the alter if necessary.
7. Change seasonings to your inclination.
8. Put aside.
9. Once the sweet potatoes are prepared, expel them from the broiler and exchange to a medium-sized bowl.
10. Add the cilantro pesto to the bowl and delicately hurl until the point that all the sweet potato 3D squares are canvassed in the pesto.
11. Store in an impenetrable, without bpa, holder in the fridge.

Turmeric and Black Peppercorn Sesame Seed Crackers

Ingredients:

- 1 ¾ - cup almond flour
- ¼ - cup nutritional yeast
- 1 - flax egg
- ½ - cup organic sesame seeds
- 1 - tablespoon organic coconut oil
- 1 - teaspoon organic ground turmeric
- ½ - teaspoon Himalayan pink salt
- ½ - teaspoon organic ground garlic
- ½ - teaspoon organic ground black pepper
- freshly ground coarse Himalayan pink salt
- freshly ground black pepper corn

Instructions:

1. Heat oven to 350 ranges.
2. Incorporate the components for the flax egg (floor flax seeds + water) to a little bowl and race to the factor that inner and out united. Set aside while your installation the straggling leftovers of the wafer mix.
3. Incorporate the remainder of the additives for the wafer blend to a medium-sized bowl and mix until the factor that interior and out joined.

4. Re-whisk the flax egg and upload it to the bowl with the wafer blend; combine the entirety till the point that the moment that it's miles in particular united. The blend must be likely soaked and fragile.
5. Change the saltine blend to a preparing skillet fixed with material paper.
6. Assemble the blend up and frame it into a ball shape, crushing it firmly and join together.
7. Utilize another bit of material paper to put over the wad of saltine blend and straighten it down, with the goal that the wafer blend is in the middle of to bits of material paper.
8. Utilize a moving pin to straighten it out to a square shape, roughly 7 x 11 in the measure.
9. Evacuate the best layer of material paper and cut the batter into little squares utilizing a pizza shaper or margarine cut.
10. Utilizing a processor, sprinkle new ground coarse Himalayan pink salt and new ground dark peppercorn over the highest point of the saltines.
11. Place the heating container in the broiler at 350 degrees for roughly 20-25 minutes, watching out for them to ensure they don't consume.
12. Take the skillet out from the stove, flip the saltines over and prepare for an extra 5 minutes, once more, watching out for them to ensure they don't consume.
13. Store in a sealed shut sans bpa compartment.

Vegan Cream of Mushroom Soup

Ingredients:

- 3 - cups water
- 3 - cups organic mushrooms
- 1 - cup organic pine nuts
- 1 - organic avocado (pitted)
- ½ - cup organic red onion
- 2 - cloves organic garlic
- 1 - teaspoon organic fresh thyme
- 1 - teaspoon Himalayan pink salt
- 1 – teaspoon organic ground black pepper

Instructions:

1. Add all fixings to a Vitamix and mix until the point that everything is all around joined.
2. Modify seasonings to your inclination.
3. Contingent upon the Vitamix show you have, you might have the capacity to utilize the "soup" or "warm" setting and mix the blend for an extra 2-3 minutes to "warm" up the soup and still keep it "crude".
4. Discretionary: Garnish with additional cut mushrooms, crisp hacked red onions or natural ground dark pepper.
5. Store in a water/air proof without bpa holder in the icebox.

Spicy Turmeric Oven-Baked Sweet Potato Fries

Ingredients:

- 1 - large organic sweet potato
- 1 - tablespoon 100% pure avocado oil
- ½ - teaspoon organic turmeric powder
- ½ - teaspoon organic cayenne pepper
- ½ - teaspoon organic ground black pepper
- ½ - teaspoon Himalayan pink salt
- 2 - tablespoons nutritional yeast

Instructions:

1. Peel the skin off the sweet potato. Cut the closures off then cut it down the center through and through.
2. Cut the potato into long "French sear" pieces. You ought to have around 50-60 from an big sweet potato.
3. Include the slice sweet potato pieces to a vast blending dish.
4. Include the avocado oil and hurl the sweet potatoes until the point when the avocado oil is equitably conveyed and all pieces are secured.
5. Include every one of the elements for the flavoring to the bowl of cut sweet potatoes each one in turn (and including the nourishing yeast last) and hurl each time ensuring the seasonings are uniformly circulated and all pieces are secured before including the following flavoring.
6. Change the measure of seasonings to your inclination.

7. Place the prepared sweet potato pieces to a heating container fixed with material paper and prepare at 425 degrees for 15-20 minutes.
8. Take out the dish from the broiler, flip over every one of the fries and restore the skillet to the stove for around 5-10 more minutes. Broiler times will change, yet you need them to be marginally fresh and take mind not to consume them.
9. Best served hot from the broiler.

Classic Hummus

Ingredients:

- 1 - can Eden Organic Garbanzo Beans

- 2 - tablespoons organic tahini

- 2 - tablespoons organic lemon juice

- 2 - tablespoons organic extra-virgin olive oil

- 2 - cloves organic garlic

- ½ - teaspoon Himalayan pink salt

- 2-4 - tablespoons water (filtered/purified)

Instructions:

1. Add all fixings to a sustenance processor and process till it is rich and smooth. Begin with 2 tablespoons of water and encompass an additional 1 tablespoon more straight away at the off chance which you incline towards a narrower consistency.
2. Modify the seasonings on your inclination.
3. Garnish with additional natural chickpeas, natural ground paprika or sprinkle with herbal additional virgin olive oil. (Optional)
4. Store in a hermetically sealed sans bpa compartment in the cooler.

Oven-Baked "Fried" Artichokes

Ingredients:

- ½ - cup almond flour
- ½ - cup nutritional yeast
- ½ - teaspoon organic ground garlic
- ½ - teaspoon organic ground cayenne pepper
- ½ - teaspoon Himalayan pink salt
- can artichoke hearts (drained)
- 1 - tablespoon 100% pure avocado oil

Instructions:

1. Preheat broiler to 425 degrees.
2. Include every one of the elements for the flavoring to a little bowl and blend together until the point when all around joined. Put aside.
3. Deplete the jar of artichokes, remove the finishes, at that point cut every artichoke piece down the middle.
4. Break separated and isolate the artichoke clears out.
5. Add the artichoke pieces to a little bowl and hurl with the avocado oil until the point when they are altogether secured.
6. Sprinkle 1/2 the flavoring blend over the artichoke pieces and hurl until the point when they are altogether secured.
7. Sprinkle the other 1/2 of the flavoring blend over the artichoke pieces and hurl again until the point that they are altogether secured.

8. Change the prepared bits of artichoke to a heating skillet fixed with material paper and spread them out equally ensuring none are covering. Sprinkle any extra flavoring blend on any pieces that stay uncoated.
9. Prepare at 425 degrees for 10-15 minutes, or until brilliant darker, taking consideration not to overheat or consume them.
10. Best when served hot from the stove.

Chimichurri Sauce

Ingredients:

- 2 - cups organic fresh parsley
- 1 - cup organic fresh cilantro
- 3 - cloves organic garlic
- ¼ - cup + 1 tablespoon organic extra-virgin olive oil
- 2 - tablespoons organic apple cider vinegar
- 1 - teaspoon organic red pepper flakes
- ¼ - teaspoon Himalayan pink salt
- ½ - teaspoon organic black pepper

Instructions:

1. Add all fixings to a Vita mix and mix until the point that all around mixed and smooth, utilizing the alter if essential.
2. Change seasonings to your inclination.
3. Store in a sealed shut without bpa holder in the icebox.

Chocolate Avocado Pudding

Ingredients:

- 4 - organic avocados
- ½ - cup organic raw coconut nectar
- ¼ - cup organic raw cacao powder
- 2- teaspoon organic vanilla bean powder
- 1 - can organic full-fat coconut milk (13.5 ounce can)

Instructions:

1. Propelled readiness: Put the container of coconut drain in the cooler for 60 minutes.
2. Evacuate the container of coconut drain from the cooler. In the wake of opening the can, evacuate just the solidified part on the best 50% of the can (coconut fat) and spare the fluid part on the base of the can to make a smoothie. Try not to include the whole container of coconut drain or the fluid part to the formula.
3. Include the solidified piece of the coconut drain with the rest of the fixings to a Vitamix and mix until it's velvety and smooth.
4. Serve instantly or exchange the blend to a water/air proof sans bpa holder to chill it in the fridge before serving.
5. Store in a hermetically sealed sans bpa compartment in the icebox.

Sweet Potato Hummus

Ingredients:

- 1 - cup organic sweet potato (baked)
- ¼ - cup organic tahini
- ¼ - cup organic lime juice (freshly squeezed)
- 2 - tablespoons organic extra-virgin olive oil
- 2 - cloves organic garlic
- ½ - teaspoon organic ground black pepper
- ½ - teaspoon Himalayan pink salt

Instructions:

1. Preheat stove to 350 degrees.
2. Puncture the outside of the sweet potato with a fork on all sides.
3. Place the sweet potato on a preparing container fixed with material paper and heat for a hour.
4. Once the sweet potato is prepared, cut it down the middle, scoop out the inner parts with a spoon, and place them in a Vitamix (you ought to have +/ - 1 container heated sweet potato).
5. Include whatever remains of the fixings to the Vitamix and blend until it's smooth and smooth, using the modify if fundamental.
6. Adjust seasonings to your tendency.
7. Store in a water/air confirmation without bpa holder in the ice chest.

Lemon Dill Avocado Dressing

Ingredients:

- 2 - organic avocados (pitted)
- ¼ - cup organic lemon juice
- 1 - tablespoon organic dried dill
- 3 - cloves organic garlic
- ¼ - teaspoon organic ground black pepper
- ¼ - teaspoon Himalayan pink salt

Instructions:

1. Add all fixings to a Vitamix and mix until it is rich and clean.
2. Change seasonings for your inclination. On the off threat that you want your dressing particularly narrower, consist of 2-three teaspoons of separated/cleansed water or herbal lemon juice.
3. Store in an impenetrable sans bpa compartment in the icebox.

Raw Cacao and Raspberry Mousse Cakes

Ingredients:

For the mousse:

- ½ - cup organic freeze-dried raspberries

- ½ - cup organic hemp seeds

- ½ - cup organic raw cacao powder

- ¼ - cup organic date nectar

- ¼ - cup organic coconut oil

- ¼ - cup filtered/purified water

For the crust:

- ½ - cup almond flour

- 1/8 - cup organic date nectar

- 1/8 - cup organic coconut oil

- 1 - tablespoon organic coconut flour

- 1/8 - teaspoon organic vanilla bean powder

- 1 - pinch Himalayan pink salt

Instructions:

1. Include every one of the elements for the outside layer to a medium-sized bowl and blend until the point when all around joined.
2. Gap the covering blend uniformly between 12 smaller than usual heart shape and press it down immovably in the base of the molds. Put aside.

Prepare the mousse:

3. Include every one of the elements for the mousse (include the water and coconut oil first) to a Vitamix and mix until the point that the blend is velvety and smooth, utilizing the alter if necessary. The blend ought to be marginally thick in surface when done.
4. Separation the mousse blend uniformly between 12 smaller than usual heart forms and pour it over the outside.

Assembly:

5. Place the shape plate on a preparing container and place it in the cooler for roughly 30-a hour, or until the point when they solidify.
6. At the point when prepared to serve, expel from the cooler and let them sit on the counter for only a couple of minutes, on the off chance that they are solidified strong. Include a solitary stop dried or crisp raspberry on the best for embellish.
7. Store additional items in a hermetically sealed without bpa holder until prepared to serve since they will get delicate and lose their shape If let out at room temperature.

Chocolate Cauliflower Nice Cream Smoothie Bowl

Ingredients:

For the nice cream:

- 1 - large organic frozen banana

- 1 - cup organic frozen cauliflower rice

- ¼ - cup + 1 tablespoon homemade almond milk

- 2 - tablespoons organic raw cacao powder

- 1 - tablespoon organic almond butter

For the toppings:

- ½ - cup organic wild blueberries

- 1-2 - tablespoons organic raw cacao nibs

Instructions:

1. Include all elements for the decent cream to a Vitamix and mix on fast until the point that everything is very much consolidated and has the consistency of delicate serve dessert, utilizing the alter if necessary.
2. Change the blend to your serving bowl(s).
3. Discretionary: Top with proposed garnishes of natural wild blueberries and natural crude cacao nibs, or your most loved natural organic product or other sound fixings.

Raw No-Bake Black Forest Bars

Ingredients:

For the brownie base:

- 1 - cup organic walnuts
- 4 - organic medjool dates (pitted)
- ¼ - cup organic raw cacao powder
- 2 - tablespoon organic refined coconut oil
- 1 - pinch Himalayan pink salt

For the cherry filling:

- 1½ - cups organic cherries (pitted, halved)
- 8 - large organic medjool dates (pitted)
- 1 - tablespoon organic refined coconut oil

For the chocolate topping:

- 1 - organic avocado
- 2 - tablespoons organic refined coconut oil
- 2 - tablespoons organic raw cacao powder
- 2 - tablespoon organic date nectar
- 2 - tablespoon organic almond butter

Instructions:

Prepare the brownie base:
1. Include all elements for the brownie base to a sustenance processor and process until the point that it is all around joined and a wet, brittle blend.
2. Change the blend to a 8 x 5 heating container fixed with material paper.

3. Utilizing the back of a spoon or your hands, press the blend down solidly and uniformly in the base of the skillet. Put aside.

Prepare the cherry filling:

4. Set up the fruits: de-stem and de-seed the cherries by pulling off the stem and slicing the cherry down the middle to evacuate the pit. Place the fruits in a little bowl to quantify enough to make the formula.

5. Include every one of the elements for the cherry filling to a sustenance processor and heartbeat it 10-12 long circumstances, sufficiently long to separate the dates and fruits into lumps, taking consideration not to over process.

6. Change the cherry filling to the heating dish and spread it uniformly over the brownie base.

7. Utilizing the back of a spoon or your hands, press the blend down solidly and equally. Put aside.

Prepare the chocolate topping:

8. Include every one of the elements for the chocolate fixing to a little bowl and whisk it together until the point that it is rich and smooth and no bits of avocado remain.

9. Change the chocolate garnish to the heating skillet and spread it uniformly over the cherry filling.

Other:

10. Place the dish in the cooler for roughly 3-4 hours, or until the point that it solidifies.

11. When you are prepared to serve, expel it from the cooler and let it sit out on the ledge for only a couple of minutes so it will be less demanding to cut.

12. Store in the cooler in an impenetrable without bpa holder until prepared to serve since it will get delicate if left out at room temperature.

Vegan Raspberry and Chocolate Ice Cream Squares

Ingredients:

For the ice cream:

- 2 - organic avocados (pitted)

- 1 - can organic full-fat coconut milk (13.5 ounce can)

- ½ - cup organic raw cacao powder

- ¼ - cup organic date nectar

- ¼ - teaspoon organic vanilla bean powder

- ¼ - teaspoon Himalayan pink salt

For the add-in:

- 1 - cup organic freeze-dried raspberries

For the topping:

- ½ - cup organic freeze-dried raspberries

Instructions:

1. Propelled Preparation: Put (1) 13.5-ounce jar of full-fat coconut drain in the cooler for (1) hour preceding making this formula. You will utilize just the "fat" some portion of the coconut drain, and not the "water".
2. You can skirt this progression later on by continually keeping a container of full-fat coconut drain in the back of your icebox so it will be prepared to use immediately.
3. Take the jar of coconut drain from the cooler and evacuate just the solidified coconut "fat" part, and add

it to a Vitamix. Spare the rest of the coconut "water" from the can to use for a smoothie.

4.   Include all the rest of the elements for the frozen yogurt to the Vitamix and mix until it's velvety and smooth.

5.   Include the 1 measure of include solidify dried raspberries to the Vitamix compartment and tenderly blend them in by hand. Try not to mix them in.

6.   Change the blend to a 8 x 5 bread container fixed with material paper and spread it equitably in the skillet.

7.   Include the 1/2 measure of garnish solidify dried raspberries equitably on the highest point of the dessert blend.

8.   Put the container in the cooler for around 2-3 hours, or until the point when it solidifies.

9.   At the point when prepared to serve, expel from the cooler and cut into little square pieces or square shape bar pieces.

10. Store in a hermetically sealed without bpa holder in the cooler until prepared to serve since they will get delicate if left out at room temperature.

Vegan Dried Blueberry Protein Energy Balls

Ingredients:

- 1 - cup organic dried blueberries
- 1 - cup organic medjool dates (pitted)
- 2 - tablespoons Yuve' Vanilla Vegan Protein Powder
- 1 - tablespoon organic almond butter
- 1 - teaspoon organic vanilla bean powder

Instructions:

1. Add all fixings to a nourishment processor and heartbeat around 10 times, or sufficiently only to separate the dates into small pieces, taking consideration not to over process.
2. Take out a spoonful at any given moment, crush it in the palm of your hand, at that point move them into a ball shape.
3. Store in a hermetically sealed sans bpa holder in the icebox.

Vegan Chocolate Dipped Cherries

Ingredients:

- 14 - organic cherries
- ½ - cup Enjoy Life mini-chocolate chips
- 1 - teaspoon organic coconut oil

Instructions:

1. Put the chocolate chips and coconut oil to a little pot and dissolve on low warmth until it's clean, mixing the entire time to ensure it does not eat.
2. Delicately plunge the last 3/4 of the culmination into the softened chocolate, taking consideration to no longer sever them the stem.
3. Place the culmination on a preparing dish fixed with cloth paper and location them inside the fridge for round 15 mins, or until the factor that the chocolate solidifies.
4. Store in a hermetically sealed sans bpa holder within the icebox until prepared to serve.

Chocolate Pistachio Fudge Cups with Sea Salt

Ingredients:

For the fudge:

- 1 - cup organic pistachios
- 1 - cup organic coconut oil
- ¼ - cup organic raw cacao powder
- ¼ - cup organic date nectar
- ¼ - cup organic almond butter
- 1 - teaspoon organic vanilla bean powder

For the topping:

- Salt

Instructions:

1. Include all elements for the fudge to a medium estimated bowl and blend until the point that very much joined and smooth.
2. Partition the blend between 24 smaller than expected biscuit containers.
3. Place the scaled down biscuit glasses on a preparing sheet at that point exchange to the cooler for around 5-10 minutes, or sufficiently ache for the tops to get somewhat solidified.
4. Take the preparing sheet out from the cooler and sprinkle ocean salt over every one of the fudge

containers. In the event that the tops aren't marginally solidified from Step 3, the ocean salt will sink down into the fluid/unhardened fudge.
5.   Restore the heating dish to the cooler for around 30-a hour, or until the point when they are solidified.
6.   Store in a water/air proof sans bpa holder in the cooler or icebox until prepared to serve since they will get delicate if left out at room temperature.

Vegan Chocolate Covered Strawberry Truffles

Ingredients:

For the truffles:

- 2 - cups organic freeze-dried strawberries

- 8 - large organic medjool dates (pitted)

For the chocolate coating:

- ½ - cup Enjoy Life mini-chocolate chips*

- 1 - teaspoon organic coconut oil

Instructions:

Prepare the truffles:
1. Include all elements for the truffles to a sustenance processor and process until the point that it turns into a sticky, brittle surface.
2. Take out a little spoonful at any given moment and move them into a ball shape. Put aside.
Prepare the chocolate coating:
3. Include every one of the elements for the chocolate covering to a little sauce dish and soften on most minimal warmth, blending the whole time until the point when it ends up smooth.
Assembly:
4. Include each ball into the pan with the liquefied chocolate and delicately hurl around till the factor that they may be totally secured.
5. Take them out from the pan and area them on a plate or heating dish fixed with fabric paper.
6. Place them in the cooler for around 15-half-hour, or until the factor while the chocolate solidifies.
7. Store in an impenetrable sans bpa compartment within the cooler or fridge till organized to serve considering the fact that they may get delicate if ignored at room temperature.

Vegan "Cheesy" Broccoli Bites

Ingredients:

For the broccoli:

- 3 - cups organic broccoli florets
- 2 - tablespoons 100% pure avocado oil

For the seasoning:

- ¼ - cup almond flour
- ¼ - cup nutritional yeast
- ¼ - teaspoon organic ground garlic powder
- 1/8 - - 1/4 teaspoon organic ground cayenne pepper
- 1/4 - teaspoon Himalayan pink salt

Instructions:

1. Preheat the oven to 400 degrees.
   Prepare the seasoning:
2. Include every one of the elements for the flavoring to a little bowl and mix until the point when all around consolidated. Change seasonings to your inclination. Put aside.
   Prepare the broccoli:
3. Add the broccoli florets to an extensive bowl, at that point shower the avocado oil over the best.
4. Hurl the broccoli until the point that the avocado oil is equitably conveyed and all pieces are secured.
5. Sprinkle 1/2 the flavoring blend over the broccoli pieces and delicately hurl until the point that it's equally conveyed and all pieces are secured.

6. Place the prepared broccoli pieces on a heating dish fixed with material paper and heat at 400 degrees for roughly 10 minutes.
7. Take the skillet out from the broiler and exchange the broccoli pieces once again into the vast bowl.
8. Sprinkle the rest of the 1/2 of the flavoring blend to finish everything and delicately re-hurl until the point when it's equally conveyed and all pieces are secured.
9. Restore the heating skillet to the broiler and prepare for an extra 20-25 minutes, or until fresh.

Vegan Chilled Mixed Berry and Mint Soup

Ingredients:

For the soup:

- 1 - cup frozen organic berries:

- ½ - cup filtered/purified water

- 1 - teaspoon organic lemon juice (freshly squeezed)

- 8 - organic mint leaves (fresh)

For the sweetener:

- ¼ - cup organic coconut sugar

- ¼ - cup filtered/purified water

Instructions:

Prepare the sweetener:
1. Include the coconut sugar and separated/refined water to a little pot on low/medium warmth and blend for around 1-2 minutes, or until the point that the sugar is broken up. Permit to cool before adding to the soup blend.

Prepare the soup:
2. Include every one of the elements for the soup and the sweetener blend (after it's cooled totally) to a Vitamix and mix until the point when it is very much consolidated.
3. Strain the soup blend through a strainer to expel the seeds from the organic product (spare to add to a smoothie later!)
4. Store in a water/air proof sans bpa compartment in the cooler.

Vegan Lemon Mousse Tarts

Ingredients:

For the mousse:

- 1 -can organic full-fat coconut milk (13.5 ounce can)
- 2 - tablespoons organic lemon juice
- 2 - tablespoons organic granular sweetener

For the crust:

- ½ - cup organic raw pecans
- 2 - organic medjool dates
- ½ - tablespoon organic coconut oil
- 1/8 - teaspoon organic vanilla bean powder
- 1 - pinch Himalayan pink salt

Instructions:

1. Propelled Preparation: Add a container of natural full-fat coconut drain to the back of your fridge for no less than 12-24 hours before making this formula.
2. Set up the outside layer:
3. Include all elements for the outside layer to a sustenance processor and process until the point that all around joined a brittle.
4. Change the outside layer blend to little silicone tart molds (or silicone biscuit mugs) and press down solidly.
5. Place them in the cooler on a heating sheet while you set up the mousse.
6. Set up the mousse:

7. take the coconut drain out from the icebox and scoop out the solidified "fat" some portion of the coconut drain. The base portion of the can will be fluid (spare this coconut water to add to a smoothie!).
8. Include the solidified coconut fat, lemon juice and sweetener of your decision to a blender and blend on rapid until the point that it transforms into a cushy mousse and is sufficiently thick to "top".
9. Get together:
10. Take the tart outside layers from the cooler.
11. Fill every tart outside layer with the mousse filling, isolating it equitably between the tart coverings.
12. Serve quickly or chill them in the cooler or fridge before serving.
13. Discretionary: Garnish with finely destroyed coconut.
14. Store in a water/air proof sans bpa holder in the cooler or fridge until prepared to serve in light of the fact that the covering will get delicate and lose its shape if left out at room temperature.

Vegan Vanilla Bean Ice Cream

Ingredients:

- 2 - can full-fat organic coconut milk (13.5-ounce cans)
- ½ - cup organic granular sweetener
- 2 - teaspoons organic vanilla extract
- 1 - teaspoon organic vanilla bean powder
- 1 - pinch Himalayan pink salt

Instructions:

1. Add all fixings to a Vitamix and mix until the factor that everything is very tons joined.
2. Change the combination to your frozen yogurt machine and have an impact on the ice to cream as indicated by using your gadget bearings.
3. Once the frozen yogurt is accomplished, you could both an) admire it as delicate serve dessert or b) change the combo to a without bpa cooler safe holder, cover firmly and solidify for 2 or 3 hours, or till the point when it solidifies to the consistency of customary dessert.

Almond Butter Swirl, Chocolate Avocado Ice Cream

Ingredients:

For the ice cream:

- 1 - can organic full-fat coconut milk (13.5 ounce can)
- 2- organic avocados (pitted)
- ¼ - cup organic raw cacao powder
- ¼ - ½ - cup non-GMO xylitol

For the swirl:

- ½- cup organic almond butter
- 1 - tablespoon organic date nectar

Instructions:

Prepare the ice cream:
1. Include all elements for the dessert to a Vitamix and mix until it's rich and smooth. Alter the measure of sweetener to your inclination.
2. Change the blend to a dessert creator and process as per your machines headings.

Prepare the swirl:
3. Include every one of the elements for the whirl to a little bowl and blend until the point when very much joined. Put aside.

Assemble:
4. At the point when the frozen yogurt creator is done influencing the ice to cream, exchange the blend to a

water/air proof sans bpa, cooler safe dessert compartment and spread equitably.
5. The kind of almond spread you utilize will figure out which choice to utilize:
6. Choice 1: If your twirl blend is thin, drop a spoonful of the whirl over the frozen yogurt and utilizing the tip of a sharp blade, whirl it into the dessert blend.
7. Alternative 2: If your whirl blend is thick, take out a little sum at any given moment and move it into little balls (you ought to have +/ - 30 modest balls). Drop the balls into the frozen yogurt blend, spreading them equitably then drive them down into the dessert with a fork or level edged spoon.
8. Cover your compartment and place in the cooler for 2-3 hours, or until the point that it gets to the hardness you lean toward.

Vegan Strawberry Mousse

Ingredients:

- 1 - can organic full-fat coconut milk (13.5 ounce can)

- 3 - tablespoons organic freeze-dried strawberries

- 2 - tablespoons organic unrefined granular sweetener

Instructions:

1. Moved Preparation: Add a holder of characteristic full-fat coconut deplete to the back of your refrigerator no under 12-24 hours before making this equation.
2. Once the coconut deplete has been refrigerated no under 12-24 hours, remove the can from the cooler. Open the can and scoop out the cemented "fat" a few
3. portion of the coconut drain from the best 50% of the can. The base half will be fluid (spare this coconut water to add to a smoothie!).
4. Include the solidified coconut fat, granular sweetener or xylitol, and solidify dried strawberries to a blender and blend on fast until the point when it transforms into a cushioned mousse and sufficiently thick to "top". Alter the sweetener to your inclination.
5. Serve quickly or store in the cooler in a sealed shut without bpa holder since it will get delicate if left out at room temperature.
6. Discretionary: Top with natural destroyed coconut drops.

Healthy Honey Mustard Dressing

Ingredients:

- ½ - cup organic Dijon mustard
- ¼ - cup organic raw honey
- 2 - tablespoons organic extra virgin olive oil

Instructions:

1. Add all fixings to a medium-sized bowl and whisk together until the point when all around mixed and smooth in surface.
2. Alter sweetener to your inclination.
3. Store in the fridge in a water/air proof, without bpa holder.

Vegan Chocolate Covered Turtles

Ingredients:

For the caramel mixture:

- 1½ - cups organic medjool dates (pitted)
- 2 - tablespoons organic almond butter
- 2 - tablespoons water (filtered/purified)
- 1 - tablespoon organic coconut oil
- 1 - pinch Himalayan pink salt

For the mix-in:

- 1 - cup organic pecans (chopped)

For the chocolate coating:

- 1 - cup Enjoy Life mini-chocolate chips
- 1 - tablespoons organic coconut oil

Instructions:

Prepare the caramel mixture:

1. Include all elements for the caramel blend to a Vitamix and mix on "high" speed until the point when it turns into a thick, pale write consistency. You may need to stop and rub the sides a few times.
2. Change the caramel blend to a medium measured bowl and include the hacked pecans. Delicately blend in until the point when they are uniformly appropriated.
3. Take out a spoonful at any given moment, delicately move them into the palms of your hands into a ball

shape and after that tenderly press them down into a level plate shape. Put aside.

Prepare the chocolate coating:

4. Include the elements for the chocolate fixing to a little pot and dissolve on the least warmth setting, blending until the point that it is softened and smooth and taking consideration not to consume it.

Assembly:

5. Take each turtle and delicately put it in the pot with the liquefied chocolate and utilize a fork to tenderly flip it over to coat the opposite side.
6. Lift each turtle out of the chocolate blend with a fork underneath it, giving the overabundance chocolate a chance to trickle off before moving it to the preparing sheet.
7. Change the chocolate secured turtles to a preparing sheet fixed with material paper.
8. Place them in the cooler for roughly 30 - a hour, or until the point when they end up solidified.
9. Store in the cooler in an impermeable sans bpa holder until the point when you are prepared to serve since they will get delicate and lose their shape at room temperature.

Vegan Tahini Brownie Truffles

Ingredients:

For the truffles:

- 1 - cup organic medjool dates (pitted)
- ½ - cup organic tahini
- ½ - cup almond flour
- ¼ - cup organic raw cacao powder
- 2 -tablespoons homemade almond milk
- ½ - teaspoon organic vanilla bean powder
- 1 - pinch Himalayan pink salt

For the coating:

- ¼ - cup organic raw cacao powder
- ¼ - cup organic date nectar
- ¼ - cup organic coconut oil

For the topping:

- ¼ - cup organic walnuts (chopped)

Instructions:

1. Include every one of the elements for the truffles to a nourishment processor and process until the point that it turns into a wet, brittle surface.
2. Take out a spoonful at any given moment and move it into a ball shape between the palms of your hands.

3. Put the truffles on a heating dish fixed with material paper in the cooler to firm while you set up the covering.
4. Include every one of the elements for the covering to a little pot and soften on most minimal warmth, mixing until the point when it's very much joined and smooth, and taking consideration not to consume it.
5. Take out from stove best and permit to cool.
6. Once the covering has cooled, expel the skillet of truffles from the cooler and take every truffle and delicately move it into the covering blend, ensuring it's totally secured.
7. Place the covered truffles back on the heating skillet fixed with material paper.
8. Discretionary: Sprinkle hacked walnuts over the truffles.
9. Put the preparing skillet back in the cooler for around 15 minutes to enable the covering to solidify.
10. Store in a water/air proof, without bpa holder in the cooler or fridge until prepared to serve since they will get delicate if left out at room temperature.

Vegan Taco "Meat"

Ingredients:

- 2 - cups organic walnuts
- 10 - teaspoons organic extra-virgin olive oil
- ½ - teaspoon Himalayan pink salt
- 1 - teaspoon organic cumin powder
- 1 - teaspoon organic chipotle powder
- 1 - teaspoon organic chili powder

Instructions:

1. Add all fixings to a sustenance processor and process it till the separated into minor pieces, and pay attention so as not to over process.
2. Change seasonings to your tendency.
3. Use as a topping on nachos or as filling for taco, wrap, and baked sweet potato, avocado, salad, etc.
4. Store in an air-tight BPA-free container in the refrigerator.

Vegan Chocolate Avocado Frosting

Ingredients:

- 2 - organic avocados
- ¼ - cup organic raw cacao powder
- ¼ - cup organic almond butter
- ¼ - cup organic date nectar
- 1 - 2 - pinches Himalayan pink salt

Instructions:

1. Add the avocados to a little bowl and whisk together until the point when they are velvety and totally smooth, with no modest pieces.
2. Include the rest of the fixings and whisk everything together until the point that it is velvety, thick and smooth.
3. Use as you would in any formula that calls for "chocolate icing".
4. Discretionary: If you lean toward the icing to be thicker, simply placed it in the icebox for around 15-30 minutes and it will thicken up.

Vegan Cacao Almond Balls

Ingredients:

- 1 - cup organic raw almonds
- ½ - cup organic almond butter
- ¼ - cup almond flour
- ¼ - cup organic raw cacao powder
- 2 - tablespoons organic hemp oil
- 2 - tablespoons organic maca powder
- 1 - tablespoon organic date nectar
- ½ - teaspoon organic vanilla bean powder

Instructions:

1. Add all fixings to a nourishment processor and process until the point when everything is all around consolidated and it has a thick glue write consistency. Don't over process the almonds, they ought to be in minor pieces.
2. Modify the sweetener to your inclination.
3. Take out a spoonful at any given moment and move it between the palms of your hands to influence a ball to shape.
4. Refrigerate until prepared to serve to keep them firm.
5. Store in an impenetrable without bpa holder.

Vegan Caramel Sauce

Ingredients:

- ½ - cup organic almond butter
- ½ - cup organic coconut oil
- ½ - cup organic maple syrup
- ½ - teaspoon organic vanilla bean powder
- 1/8 - teaspoon Himalayan pink salt

Instructions:

1. Add all fixings to a little bowl and whisk together with a rush until it's rich and smooth and everything is all around consolidated, particularly the coconut oil.
2. Store in the wash room or icebox in a hermetically sealed sans bpa compartment. In the event that you store it in the fridge, it will turn out to be thick and possibly strong because of the coconut oil. Simply run your compartment under warm water to soften it again and re-blend.

Vegan Cilantro and Lime Cauliflower Rice

Ingredients:

For the cauliflower rice:

- 2 - cups organic cauliflower rice

- 2 - tablespoons organic lime juice

- 1 - tablespoon 100% pure avocado oil

- 1 - teaspoon Himalayan pink salt

- ½ - teaspoon organic ground black pepper

For the add-in:

- ¼ - cup organic fresh cilantro (chopped)

Instructions:

1. Include every one of the elements for the cauliflower rice to a skillet and gently sauté for roughly 5 minutes, or until the point when it gets to the consistency that you incline toward. Change seasonings to your inclination.
2. Take out from warmth and include the cleaved cilantro and blend until the point that it's uniformly appropriated
3. Change to your serving dish and enhancement with additional hacked cilantro.

Vegan Spinach Pesto

Ingredients:

- 2 - cups organic spinach
- ¾ - cup organic walnuts
- ½ - cup organic extra-virgin olive oil
- ½ - cup nutritional yeast
- 2 - tablespoons organic lemon juice
- ¼ - ½ - teaspoon Himalayan pink salt

Instructions:

1. Add all fixings to a Vitamix and mix until the point that everything is all around consolidated. Note: I utilized a Vitamix Professional 750 Series with a wet compartment and mixed beginning at speed 1 at that point gradually moving to speed 10, at that point gradually back to speed 1 (sufficiently long to slash the nuts and get it to a puree-type surface).
2. Change seasonings to your inclination.
3. Store in a sealed shut sans bpa holder.

Shirataki Angel Hair Pasta with Creamy Chipotle Avocado Sauce

Ingredients:

- 2 - packs Shirataki Angel Hair Pasta

For the sauce:

- 2 avocados

- ¼ - cup extra-virgin olive oil

- 2 tablespoons lime juice

- ½ - 1 - teaspoon organic ground chipotle powder

- ¼ - ½ - teaspoon Himalayan pink salt

Instructions:

1. Set up the pasta as indicated by the bearings on the bundle.
2. Include all elements for the sauce to a Vitamix and mix until it's velvety and smooth.
3. Change seasonings to your inclination.
4. Change the readied pasta noodles to a medium-sized bowl.
5. Include the sauce into the bowl with the noodles and tenderly hurl until the point when it's uniformly dispersed
6. Discretionary: Garnish with hacked natural crisp cilantro or natural child spinach.
7. Best when served warm.

Carrot Apple and Celery Juice

Ingredients:

- 4 - organic carrots
- 1 - organic apple
- 2 - stalks organic celery
- ½ - organic lemon

Instructions:

1. Wash and cut your veggies/natural product to be set up to use in your juicer.
2. Juice the carrots, apple and celery as per your juicers directions.
3. Hand-press the lemon into the juice after the various veggies/organic product have been squeezed and blend in.

Vegan Flourless "Cheesy" Garlic Breadsticks

Ingredients:

For the breadsticks:

- 2 - cups almond flour

- 2 - cups Dahiya Mozzarella Cheese

- 1 - teaspoon organic extra-virgin olive oil

- 1 - teaspoon organic ground garlic powder

- ½ - teaspoon Himalayan pink salt

- 3 - flax eggs (3 tablespoons ground flax seeds + 9 tablespoons filtered/purified water)

For the garlic topping:

- 4 - cloves organic garlic (freshly crushed)

- 1 - tablespoon organic extra-virgin olive oil

- 1 - tablespoon organic dried oregano

- 1/8 - teaspoon Himalayan pink salt

- 1/8 - teaspoon organic ground black pepper

Instructions:

1. Preheat stove to 350 degrees.
2. Set up the breadsticks:
3. Include every one of the elements for the breadsticks to a medium estimated bowl and mix until the point that very much consolidated.

4. Change the blend to a heating skillet fixed with material paper.
5. Frame the blend into a ball shape, at that point utilizing your hands, straighten it out into a square shape roughly 1/2-inch-thick and around a 8 x 8 square.
6. Heat at 350 degrees for around 15-20 minutes, or until it's brilliant on the best and edges.
7. Evacuate the broiler to include the garlic topping.
8. Set up the garlic topping:
9. Include all elements for the garlic fixing to a little bowl and blend together until the point when all around consolidated. Modify seasonings to your inclination.
10. Pour the garnish over the bread sticks and spread a thin layer equally over the best.
11. Utilize a blade or pizza shaper to cut into breadstick shapes or chomp measured pieces.
12. Best when served warm straight from the broiler.

Vegan Fresh Herb and Tahini Pesto

Ingredients:

- 1 - cup organic parsley leaves
- 1 - cup cilantro leaves
- 1 - tablespoon mint leaves
- 2 - tablespoons tahini
- 2 - tablespoons lemon juice
- 1 - tablespoon extra-virgin olive oil
- 2 - cloves garlic (freshly crushed)
- 1/8 - ¼ - teaspoon Himalayan pink salt

Instructions:

1. Add all fixings to a nourishment processor and process until the point when it is all around mixed.
2. Modify the seasonings to your inclination.

Vegan Sweet Potato and Pecan Balls

Ingredients:

- ***For the balls:***
- 1 - cup sweet potatoes (cooked)
- 1/3 - cup pecans (chopped)
- 2 - tablespoons date nectar (use code DVASH_THFH to save 15% off your order)
- 1 - 2 - teaspoons organic pumpkin pie spice
- ***For the topping:***
- 1/3 - cup organic pecans (chopped)

Instructions:

1. Heat the sweet potatoes as indicated by your favored strategy. (I jump at the chance to put mine on a heating sheet fixed with material paper and prepare at 350 degrees for around 45-a hour, or until the point that they are delicate within). Enable them to totally cool before setting off to the following stage.
2. Include the cooked sweet potatoes (after they've chilled) to a medium-sized bowl and crush them with a fork until the point when they are the consistency of "pureed potatoes".
3. Include the date nectar, pecans and pumpkin zest to the crushed sweet potatoes and mix until the point when all

around consolidated. Alter the sweetener and additionally flavors to your inclination.

4. Take out a spoonful at any given moment and delicately shape them into a ball shape. They will be to some degree delicate, however ought to have the capacity to frame the state of a ball.

5. Choice 1: Add the 1/3 measure of slashed pecans (for the garnish) to a little bowl and roll every sweet potato ball into the pecans until the point when they are secured. Tenderly search any free pecans so they don't tumble off.

6. Choice 2: Add 1-2 tablespoons of natural cinnamon + non-GMO xylitol blend to a little bowl and roll the sweet potato balls until the point when they are secured.

7. Choice 3: Leave them plain.

Chipotle Almond Stuffed Brussels Sprouts

Ingredients:

- 15 - 20 - organic brussels sprouts

For the stuffing:

- 1 - cup organic almonds

- ¼ - cup organic extra virgin olive oil

- 2 - cloves organic garlic

- 2 - tablespoons organic lemon juice

- 2 - tablespoons nutritional yeast

- 1 - tablespoon organic apple cider vinegar

- 1 - teaspoon organic ground chipotle

- ½ - teaspoon Himalayan pink salt

Instructions:

Prepare the brussels sprouts:
1. Cut the closures off all the brussels sprouts and cut them down the middle.
2. Choice 1: Raw - Set aside.
3. Choice 2: Blanched - Put them in a medium estimated pot with separated/cleansed water and rapidly whiten for 1-2 minutes or until the point when they turn brilliant green.
4. Strain and enable them to cool totally before planning to include the stuffing.

5. After they are cooled, expel the internal piece of the Brussels grows until just the external "shell" remains. Ensure you leave enough of the external piece of the brussels sprouts to help the stuffing.
    Prepare the stuffing:
6. Include every one of the elements for the stuffing to a sustenance processor and process until the point that it turns into a brittle, stout surface. Take mind not to over process, sufficiently only to separate the almonds into little pieces. Alter the seasonings to your inclination.
    Assemble:
7. Add the stuffing to the internal parts of the Brussels grows.
8. Choice 1: Eat them crude and appreciate them promptly
9. Choice 2: Sprinkle the finish with nourishing yeast and prepare at 400 degrees for roughly 20 minutes, or until the point that the tops are brilliant.

Vegan Basil Pesto and Cauliflower Rice Dip

Ingredients:

For the pesto:

- 4 - cups fresh basil
- ½ - cup walnuts
- ¼ - cup nutritional yeast
- ¼ - cup extra-virgin olive oil
- 2 - tablespoons lemon juice
- ½ - teaspoon Himalayan pink salt
- ¼ - teaspoon ground black pepper

For the cauliflower rice:

- 4 - cups organic cauliflower rice
- ½ - cup organic red onions (diced)
- 1 - tablespoon organic extra-virgin olive oil
- 2 - cloves organic garlic (freshly crushed)
- ½ - teaspoon Himalayan pink salt
- ½ - teaspoon organic ground black pepper

Instructions:

Prepare the pesto:

1. Include all elements for the pesto to a Vitamix and mix until the point when it is very much consolidated and

has a thick surface. Modify seasonings to your inclination. Put aside.

Prepare the cauliflower rice:

2. Include all elements for the cauliflower rice to a skillet and daintily sauté until the point when the onions and cauliflower are delicate.
3. Add the pesto blend to the skillet and mix until the point when everything is all around joined. Modify seasonings to your inclination.
4. Change to your serving bowl(s) and is best served hot/warm.
5. Store in a water/air proof without bpa holder in the icebox.

Vegan Chocolate Avocado Pistachio Truffles

Ingredients:

For the truffles:

- 1 - organic avocado

- 1 - cup organic medjool dates

- ½ - cup organic almond butter

- 2 - tablespoons organic raw cacao powder

- 1 - tablespoon organic coconut oil

- 1 - tablespoon filtered/purified water

- 1/8 - teaspoon organic vanilla bean powder

- 1 - pinch Himalayan pink salt

For the add-in:

- ¼ - cup organic pistachios (chopped)

For the coating:

- ¼ - cup organic pistachios (ground)

Instructions:

Prepare the pistachios:

1. For the include ins: Chop the pistachios into little pieces utilizing the level side of a spread blade. Put aside.
2. For the covering: Add the pistachios to an espresso processor and granulate them into a powder. Exchange to a little bowl. Put aside.

Prepare the truffles:

3. Include all elements for the truffles to a sustenance processor and process until the point that it shapes a thick ball. It ought to be soggy and wet.
4. Include the slashed pistachios and blend in by hand until the point when they are equitably conveyed.
5. Take out a spoonful at any given moment and move into a ball shape between the palms of your hands.
6. Add every truffle to the bowl of ground pistachios and tenderly hurl until the point that the whole truffle is secured.
7. Place the covered truffles on a plate fixed with material paper.
8. Appreciate quickly or put In the fridge for 10-15 minutes to firm.
9. Store in a sans bpa impenetrable holder.

Vegan Pecan Pie Truffles

Ingredients:

- 1 - cup organic pecans
- 8 - organic medjool dates (pitted)
- ½ - teaspoon organic vanilla bean powder

Instructions:

1. Add all fixings to a nourishment processor and process until the point that it turns into a brittle, sticky surface.
2. Take out a spoonful at any given moment and press the blend firmly with your clench hand to conservative it, at that point move it into the state of a ball with the palms of your hands.
3. Appreciate promptly or put them in the icebox for around 10-15 minutes to firm.
4. Store in a without bpa hermetically sealed holder.

Vegan Cream of Asparagus Soup

Ingredients:

For the sautéed veggies:

- 12 - stalks organic asparagus

- 1 - cup organic onion (diced)

- 3 - cloves organic garlic (freshly crushed)

- 2 - teaspoons organic extra-virgin olive oil

- ½ - 1 - teaspoon Himalayan pink salt

- ½ - 1 - teaspoon organic ground pepper

For the add-ins:

- 1 - cup organic vegetable broth

- 1 - can organic full-fat coconut milk (13.5 ounce can)

Instructions:

Prepare the veggies:
1. Cut both the onions and asparagus into small pieces.
Prepare the sautéed veggies:
2. Include the asparagus, onions, garlic, olive oil, Himalayan pink salt and dark pepper to a skillet and sauté on medium-high warmth until the point that the onions and asparagus turn out to be delicate. Change the seasonings to your inclination.
Prepare the soup:
3. Include the vegetable soup and whole jar of coconut drain to a Vitamix.

4. Include the sautéed veggie mixture high-quality of the fluids in the Vitamix.
5. Mix on "high" or the "soup" placing (in the event that you have a version with pre-custom designed settings) and mix until it is wealthy and smooth.
6. Warm it at the range pinnacle or at the "soup" putting of your Vitamix.

Conclusions

While lectins may cause some harm, there is solid research to help the advantages of eating plant nourishments.

Numerous plants are high in lectins, yet lectin levels can contrast fundamentally between plant composes. There are additionally numerous sorts of lectins, and some appear to be gainful.

It is additionally vital to know that a great part of the exploration on lectins has been through creature or test-tube examines. Moreover, numerous examinations have taken a gander at single lectins rather than the nourishments that contain them.

More research is required before following a sans lectin eating regimen can be suggested. As of now, it is by all accounts to a greater degree a pattern than an arrangement upheld by science.

www.ingramcontent.com/pod-product-compliance
Lightning Source LLC
Chambersburg PA
CBHW051307250726
48656CB00004B/1522